D1366435

HEADACHE THROUGH THE AGES

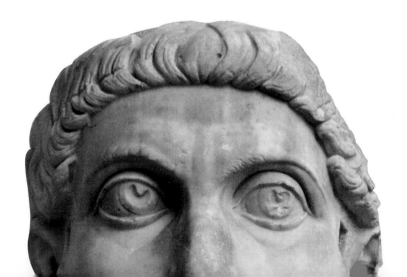

PROFESSIONAL
COMMUNICATIONS, INC.
A Medical Publishing Company

Marketing Office:
400 Center Bay Drive
West Islip, NY 11795
(t) 631/661-2852
(f) 631/661-2167

Editorial Office:
PO Box 10
Caddo, OK 74729-0010
(t) 580/367-9838
(f) 580/367-9989

For orders only, please call
1-800-337-9838
or visit our website at
www.pcibooks.com

ISBN: 1-932610-06-5

Printed in the United States of America

DISCLAIMER

The opinions expressed in this publication reflect those of the authors. However, the authors make no warranty regarding the contents of the publication. The protocols described herein are general and may not apply to a specific patient. Any product mentioned in this publication should be taken in accordance with the prescribing information provided by the manufacturer.

This text is printed on recycled paper.

TABLE OF CONTENTS

HISTORICAL VIEW...8

1. INTRODUCTION...9

2. THE ANCIENTS' VIEW OF HEADACHE AND PAIN...12

3. HEADACHE IN THE BIBLE AND TALMUD...29

4. HEADACHE IN THE MIDDLE AGES...34

5. HEADACHE IN THE RENAISSANCE...51

6. HEADACHE IN THE 17TH CENTURY...57

HEADACHE TYPES AND NOTABLE
PEOPLE AFFECTED BY THEM
THROUGH THE 20TH CENTURY...63

7. MIGRAINE...65

a. Migraine Pathogenesis...66

b. Clinical Features of Migraine...68

c. The Migraine Prodrome...77

d. Migraine Personality...87

e. Migraine Triggers...94

f. Complicated Migraine...96

8. CLUSTER HEADACHES...100

a. Clinical Features...101

b. Cluster Variants...106

9. TENSION-TYPE HEADACHES...107

10. HEADACHE TREATMENT —
A HISTORICAL PERSPECTIVE...114

CONCLUSION...126

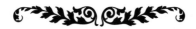

HISTORICAL VIEW

INTRODUCTION

FROM THE BOOK OF GENESIS: GOD SAID, "IT IS NOT GOOD THAT THE MAN SHOULD BE ALONE. I WILL MAKE HIM A HELP-MATE".... SO YAHWEH GOD MADE THE MAN FALL INTO A DEEP SLEEP. AND WHILE HE SLEPT, HE TOOK ONE OF HIS RIBS AND ENCLOSED IT IN FLESH. YAHWEH GOD BUILT THE RIB HE HAD TAKEN FROM THE MAN INTO A WOMAN, AND BROUGHT HER TO THE MAN. THAT NIGHT, THE FIRST MAN, ADAM, AND THE FIRST WOMAN, EVE, SPENT THEIR FIRST NIGHT TOGETHER IN THE GARDEN OF EDEN ... AND THE NEXT MORNING, THE MAN LOOKED UP TO GOD AND SAID,

"WHAT IS A HEADACHE?"

FIGURE 1: Adam & Eve. Circa 1650, Eve offers Adam the fruit of the tree of knowledge of good and evil in the garden of Eden. Original Artwork: "Theatrum Biblicum" by Johann Fischen (circa 1650). Credit Line: Hulton Archive/Getty Images

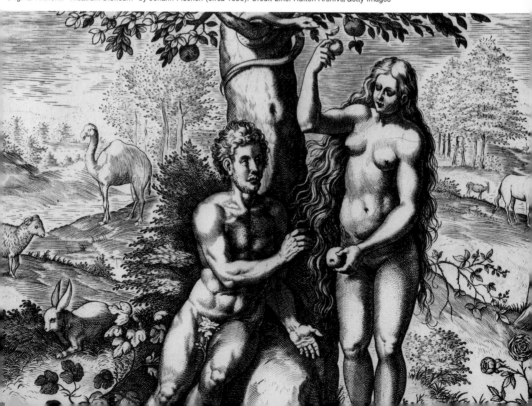

INTRODUCTION

e thought this parody would serve as a fitting beginning to this book which will explore the historical and illustrative features of headache as it has been depicted in both the arts and literature thoughout the ages. Although headache does not date back to Genesis, it does have ancient roots throughout human history. Cephalalgia has been described in literature, history, art, song, theater, and religion. It has been the subject of much over-labored humor. One anecdote about George Bernard Shaw, the eminent Anglo-Irish playwright and critic, aptly introduces the significance of the subject of this text. At a social gathering, Shaw had the opportunity to meet Friedtjof Nansen, the Norwegian arctic explorer, as well as the winner of the Nobel Peace Prize in 1922 for his relief efforts following World War I:

ABOUT ONCE A MONTH, UNTIL THE AGE OF 70 YEARS,
GEORGE BERNARD SHAW SUFFERED A DEVASTATING HEADACHE
WHICH LASTED FOR A DAY. ONE AFTERNOON, AFTER RECOVERING
FROM AN ATTACK, HE WAS INTRODUCED TO NANSEN AND ASKED
THE FAMOUS ARCTIC EXPLORER WHETHER HE HAD EVER DISCOVERED
A HEADACHE CURE. "NO," SAID NANSEN WITH A LOOK OF AMAZE-
MENT. "HAVE YOU EVER TRIED TO FIND A CURE FOR HEADACHES?"
"NO." "WELL, THAT IS A MOST ASTONISHING THING," EXCLAIMED SHAW.
"YOU HAVE SPENT YOUR LIFE IN TRYING TO DISCOVER THE NORTH
POLE, WHICH NOBODY ON EARTH CARES TUPPENCE ABOUT, AND YOU
HAVE NEVER ATTEMPTED TO DISCOVER A CURE FOR THE HEADACHE,
WHICH EVERY LIVING PERSON IS CRYING ALOUD FOR."

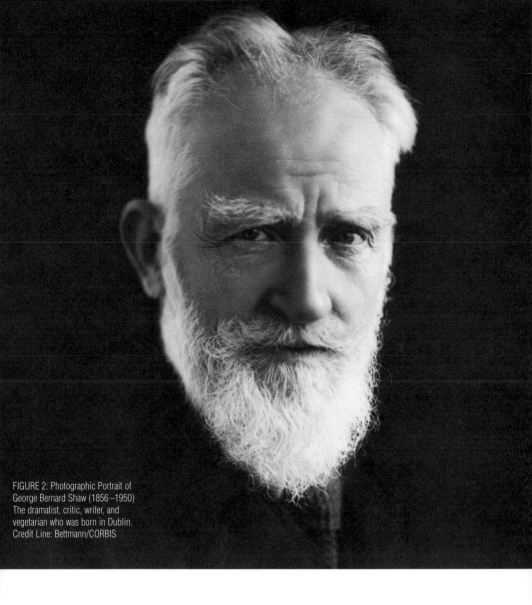

FIGURE 2: Photographic Portrait of
George Bernard Shaw (1856–1950)
The dramatist, critic, writer, and
vegetarian who was born in Dublin.
Credit Line: Bettmann/CORBIS

Headache is a universal plague. It strikes virtually everybody at some time in his or her life. Many gifted sufferers throughout the years have documented "their pain" in their particular area of the arts and history. Throughout this evolution of time, we will document significant descriptions, historical notes, and references, in headache.

eadache is a malady that has existed since earliest recorded history and throughout all civilizations on earth. It is unique in that the symptoms are almost totally subjective and there is no animal role model in which we can conduct research to simulate the human sufferer, although the pathophysiology and classification of headache is still being actively debated amongst researchers and physicians. The history of headache is rich with theories, treatments, and recognition of its complexities. The earliest recorded description of headache dates to Mesopotamia in 4000 B.C. Mesopotamia refers to the region between the Tigris and Euphrates rivers in western Asia. This region was believed to have been settled about 10,000 B.C. The people of Mesopotamia evolved from the hunter-gatherer culture to a culture based on husbandry, agriculture, and permanent settlement. The southern area, known as Babylonia, is known for its leaders such as Hammurabi who established a code of laws. Northern Mesopotamia eventually became Assyria. Trade with other regions flourished that eventually opened them to conquest from other nations, including the Persians, Greeks, and then the Muslim Arabs. Modern day Iraq encompasses ancient Mesopotamia. The ancient people of Mesopotamia were afflicted with headaches and attributed their pain to Tiu, the evil spirit of headache, who supposedly attacked a victim.

DETAIL MAP OF MESOPOTAMIA

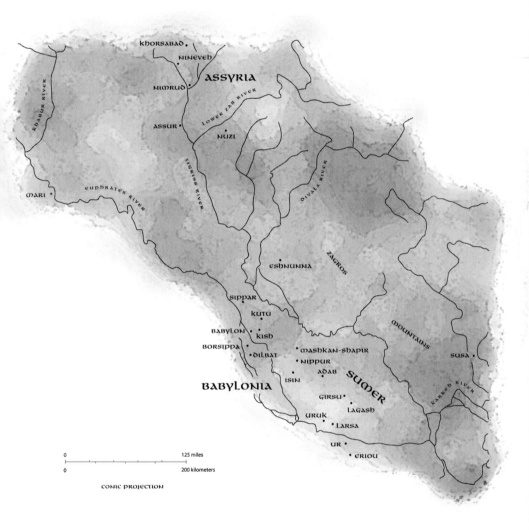

FIGURE 3: Ancient Mesopotamia

Headache roameth over the desert, blowing like the wind.
Flashing like lightning, it is loosed above and below.
It cutteth off like a reed him who feareth not his god
Like a stalk of henna, it slitteth his thews.
It wasteth the flesh of him who hath no protecting goddess.
Flashing like a heavenly star, it commeth like the dew;
It standeth hostile against the wayfarer, scorching him like the day.
This man it hath struck and
Like one with heart disease he staggereth.
Like one bereft of reason he is broken.

Migraine is a recurrent, periodic type of headache. It usually occurs one to four times per month, and will last 4 to 72 hours. The pain of migraine almost always occurs on only one side of the head, and has been described as throbbing or pulsating. The severity of a migraine attack ranges from moderate to severe, and can be incapacitating. Migraine has been described as a "sick headache," and the headache is often accompanied by nausea, vomiting, and sensitivity to light and sound. Other associated symptoms include diarrhea, fatigue, lightheadedness, sensitivity to odors, fluid retention, cold sensations in the extremities, difficulty in concentrating or memory, and dizziness. Two types of migraine headache have been classified — migraine with aura and migraine without aura. The aura usually occurs 2 to 30 minutes before the onset of the headache. Typically, the aura symptoms will be visual in nature

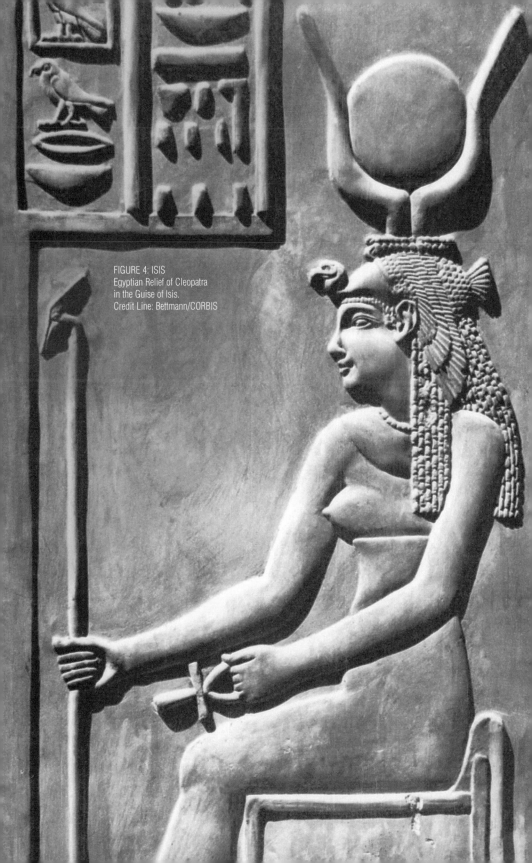

FIGURE 4: ISIS
Egyptian Relief of Cleopatra
in the Guise of Isis.
Credit Line: Bettmann/CORBIS

— the migraine sufferer seeing flashing lights, visual hallucinations, or a blind spot before the actual pain of the headache. Twenty to 30 percent of migraine sufferers will experience the symptoms of an aura with one or more attacks during their migraine history. Descriptions of the aura date back to at least the year 3000 B.C. when a Sumerian poet described a Garden of Eden called the "land of Dilmun" where:

The sick eyed says not "I am sick eyed."
The sick-headed (says) not, "I am sick-headed."

The ancient Egyptians reported their own experience with headaches. A great deal of our knowledge about their diseases and their management has been excerpted from the Ebers papyrus, a compilation of Egyptian medical texts dated about 1550 B.C. The scroll contains about 700 magical formulas and old remedies intended to cure numerous afflictions from crocodile bite to toenail pain. Remedies listed on the papyrus include: an onion crushed in honey and taken in beer; a poultice of chopped bat, wasp dung, and fresh milk; and, an application of a poultice containing a fragment of lead mixed with cat and dog dung. The Egyptians used the information on the scroll to help eliminate the house of pests (flies, rats, and scorpions). The papyrus contains an astonishingly accurate description of the circulatory system — noting the presence of blood vessels throughout the body and the heart as center of the blood supply. The papyrus was acquired by George Ebers, a German Egyptologist and novelist, in 1873. This particular quote from the Ebers papyrus includes a herbal treatment for King Usaphais' headache:

COMBINE FRANKINCENSE, CUMIN, ULAN BERRY
(UNIDENTIFIED) AND GOOSE GREASE; BOIL THESE SUBSTANCES
TOGETHER AND APPLY EXTERNALLY TO THE HEAD.

The first written reference to the central nervous system and brain dates from the Ebers papyrus. The treatment proposed for "warmth in the head" consisted of the application of moistened mortar to the head. Egyptian mythology spoke of a headache remedy used by Isis to treat Ra's headache — a combination of coriander, wormwood, juniper, honey, and opium. To the Egyptians, headache was believed to be caused by the possession of evil spirits. In the Ebers papyrus, a remedy is noted for an inflammatory condition: *"When you examine a man with an irregular wound... and that wound is inflamed... {there is} a concentration of heat: the lips of that wound are reddened and that man is hot inconsequence... then you must make cooling substances for him to draw the heat out... leaves of the willow."*

Willow bark is the forerunner of salicyclic acid — its use eventually led to the discovery of aspirin. The Assyrians recorded on stone tablets their use of willow leaves to relieve inflammatory rheumatoid disorders.[2] The Egyptians described the pain relieving effects of a concoction of myrtle or willow leaves for joint pain. The "Father of Medicine," Hippocrates, is believed to have lived on the island of Cos in ancient Greece during the 4th and 5th centuries B.C. He is best known for the Hippocratic oath, taken universally by medical students upon graduation, a document which establishes the obligations, ideals, and ethics of physicians. Aristotle in his *Politics*, called Hippocrates the "Great Physician." In approximately 460 B.C., Hippocrates described classical migraine with aura: *Most of the time he seemed to see something shining before him like a light, usually in part of the right eye, at the end of a moment, a violent pain supervened in the right temple, then in all the head and neck... vomiting when it became possible, was able to divert the pain and render it more moderate.*

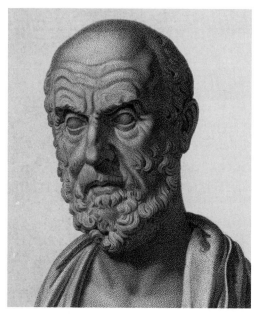

FIGURE 5: Hippocrates
Greek physician of ancient Greece,
known as the "Father of Medicine."
Credit Line: CORBIS

Hippocrates espoused the humoral theory of disease — that diseases were caused by changes in the four humors: blood, phlegm, black bile (melancholy), and yellow bile (choler). The associated symptoms of migraine, such as nausea and vomiting, were attributed to an excess of yellow bile. Hippocrates also favored the extract of willow bark to treat head pain.

The teachings of Hippocrates became universally accepted in the ancient world, and influenced generations of Greek and Roman physicians. The Greeks developed a great center of medical education and practice at Alexandria, Egypt. After their conquest, the Romans maintained this center. One ancient physician, probably trained at Alexandria, was Aretaeus of Cappodocia (A.D. 30 to 90). Very little is known about Aretaeus except he left Alexandria for Rome, and was clearly inspired by Hippocrates. Aretaeus adhered to the pneumatic school of medicine that believed that health was maintained by "vital air" or *pneuma*. Pneumatists believed that an imbalance of the four humors of Hippocrates disturbed the *pneuma*. These disturbances were manifested by an abnormal pulse. Aretaeus provided model descriptions of pleurisy, diphtheria, tetanus, pneumonia, asthma, and epilepsy. He gave diabetes its name from the Greek word for "siphon" due to the excessive thirst and urinary output of those afflicted with this disorder.

He developed the first true description of migraine as an entity distinct from the broad category of headache. He classified migraine because of its one-sidedness, association with nausea, regular recurrence, and the sequence of paroxysms of pain separated by pain-free intervals. Because the pain was unilateral, Aretaeus called this type of headache *Heterocrania*.

We now use the word, "hemicrania," meaning half-a-head. Aretaeus also distinguished between acute headache attacks lasting for days — *cephalalgia*, from chronic headache — *cephalea*.

... *But in certain cases, the parts of the right side, or those on the left solely the pain does not pass this limit, but remains in the half of the head. This is called heterocrania, an illness by no means mild... if at any time it sets in acutely, it occasions unseemly and dreadful symptoms... nausea, vomiting of bilious matters, collapse of the patient, but if... it becomes chronic, there is much torpor, heaviness of the head, anxiety and weariness. They flee the light, the darkness soothes their disease; nor can they bear readily to look upon or hear anything disagreeable; their sense of smell is vitiated. Neither does any thing agreeable to smell delight them, and they also have an aversion to fetid things; the patients, moreover, are weary of life, and wish to die... The cause of these symptoms is coldness with dryness...*

Aretaeus advocated counterirritation as the treatment of headache. He proposed that blisters should be applied to the shaved head. The blistering agents that were used included pitch, lemnestis, euphorbium, peilitory, or the juice of the thapsia.

One physician trained in Hippocratic medicine was Claudius Galen (A.D. 131 to 201), who became the most renowned physician in ancient Rome. He was born in Pergamum in Asia Minor, the site of a school of medicine. Galen is considered the founder of experimental physiology. His reputation as a great healer led him to Rome, and in 168, the emperor, Marcus Aurelius, appointed Galen physician to his son and heir, Commodus.

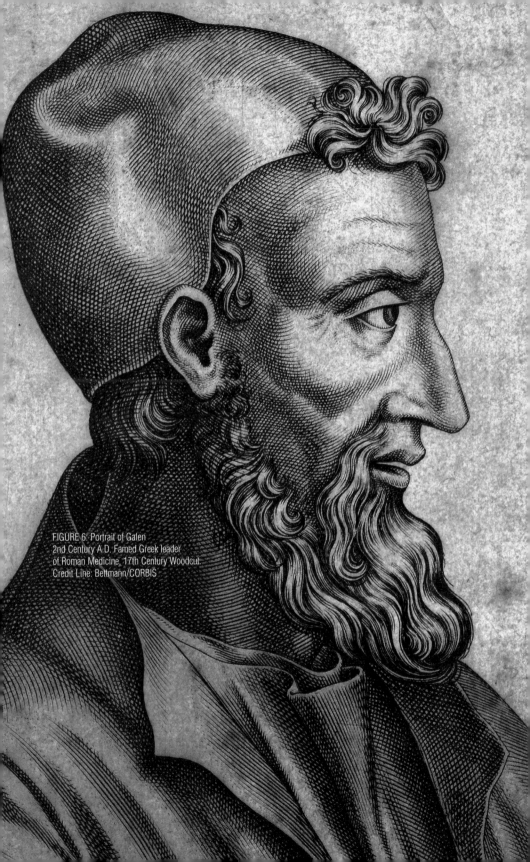

FIGURE 6: Portrait of Galen
2nd Century A.D. Famed Greek leader
of Roman Medicine, 17th Century Woodcut.
Credit Line: Bettmann/CORBIS

Via his position as a royal physician, Galen was afforded the opportunity to research and write. During the Middle Ages, Galen's texts were translated by Arab scholars, and found their way into Latin versions. His writings are believed to have influenced the emergence of science in Europe during the Renaissance.

Galen expanded on the four-humor theory by proposing that life could be attributed to three spirits, produced in the heart; and, animal spirits, which evolved from the brain. Although his erroneous theories impacted on the progress of medicine for many centuries, he did correct the Greek theory that arteries contained air instead of blood. Galen coined the term *Hemicrania*, which later became migraine. The Romans translated Hemicrania into the Latin *Hemicranium*. It was later corrupted in low Latin as Hemigranea, which became by successive abbreviations, *migranea, Migrainea*, and *Migrana*. The French modified "migrana" to *migraine*, the term now universally accepted.

❧

EACH OF THESE AFFECTIONS IS A PERMANENT PAIN OF THE HEAD, LIABLE TO BE INCREASED BY NOISES, CRIES, A BRILLIANT LIGHT, DRINKING OF WINE OR STRONG-SMELLING THINGS WHICH FILL THE HEAD. SOME FEEL AS IF THE WHOLE HEAD WERE STRUCK AND SOME AS IF ONE HALF, IN WHICH CASE THE COMPLAINT IS CALLED HEMICRANIA. WHEN THE AFFECTION IS SEATED WITHIN THE SKULL, THE PAIN EXTENDS TO THE ROOTS OF THE EYES, AND WHEN EXTERNALLY IT SPREADS AROUND THE SKULL.

❦

Galen proposed that headache was caused by a disturbance in the parts of the body that dispatch vapors or liquids containing harmful properties to the brain. He was concerned with the anatomical connections between extra- and intracranial circulation through which vapors and humors excessively fill the head.

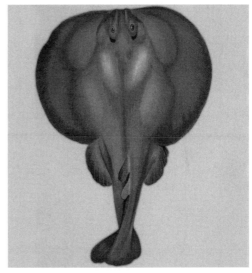

FIGURE 7: Torpedo Ray
Engraving from "A History of The Fishes" by Jonathan Couch.
Credit Line: Time Life Pictures/Getty Images

Galen also advocated counterirritation, suggesting the application of the electric torpedo fish to the forehead:

WHEN APPLIED TO THE HEAD, WHILE STILL ALIVE, IN CASES
OF HEADACHE, IT PROCURES RELIEF TO THE PAIN, PROBABLY BY ITS
PECULIAR PROPERTY OF PRODUCING TORPOR AND THE OIL OF
WHICH THE LIVING ANIMAL HAS BEEN BOILED, WHEN RUBBED IN
ALLAYS THE MOST VIOLENT PAINS OF THE JOINTS

This use of counterirritation was a precursor to the electrotherapy started by Duchenne and the transcutaneous electrical nerve stimulators (TENS) for chronic pain. Guillaume-

Benjamin-Amand Duchenne (1806 to 1875) was a French neurologist who was the first to describe several nervous and muscular disorders.

Recently, many types of chronic pain have been treated with both spinal cord electrical stimulation and TENS. TENS involves the production and transmission of electrical energy from the surface of the skin to the nervous system. The rationale for this therapy is the process by which the small, uncovered pain fibers can be controlled by the larger, covered fibers — thus reducing pain. It is sometimes described as the "gate theory" of pain. The control of these fibers will manage pain symptoms. Its efficacy has been demonstrated in conditions such as phantom pain, chronic back disorders, and headache.

Aurelius Cornelius Celsus (25 B.C. to A.D. 50) was the physician to the Emperors Tiberius and Caligula. He was the first to indicate that migraine was a lifelong nonfatal disorder, that there were trigger factors, and also emphasized that the headache would be localized or generalized.

Soranus of Ephesus (A.D. 90 to 138) trained in the Alexandrian School and worked in Rome during the reigns of Trajan and Hadrian. He was well known for his writings on obstetrics but he was also a prolific writer on acute and chronic disorders. Those in the original Greek on nervous conditions were lost, but the Latin translations of his work by Coelius Aurelianus have survived. Physicians will often hear headache patients remark: "I wake with a headache but I am not sure whether it is an ordinary headache or the beginning of a migraine." This problem was recognized by Soranus who advised his patients:

"Sit, put the head between the knees:
if the pain increased, a migraine had begun."

Soranus described scotoma which he considered as a precursor of an epileptic attack. Although the term scotoma nowadays implies a blind area in the visual field, a more accurate rendering would be a dizzy spell. This would more rationally explain why it was thought by Soranus to be a warning of an epileptic attack. For many years, epilepsy and migraine were thought to be part of the same disease process. Migraine in fact was often classified as a form of convulsive disorder, perhaps suggested by its periodicity. Today, most headache researchers recognize that there is no relationship between these two diseases.

Coelius Aurelianus was a famous physician in 5th century A.D. Tunisia and probably practiced in Rome. Among Greco-Roman physicians, he was considered second only to Galen. In his main work, *De morbis acutis et chronicis*, he emphasized the importance of accurate diagnosis and nondrug therapies. In regards to headache, he described *"the sudden fogging of vision (nebula), the lines (tractus) resembling the veins in marble called sparks (marmarygae) by the Greeks."* In a chapter entitled De Capitis Passione, he adds to unilateral headache and vomiting, vertigo, tinnitus, and deafness, so that he may have confused migraine with Ménière's Syndrome. In this chapter, he called the temporal pounding headache *crotophon*, but this term has been rarely used. Many headache researchers and clinicians consider vertigo as a prominent feature of migraine.

Alexander Trallianus (A.D. 525 to ca. 605) came from Tralles, Lydia (now called Guzel Hissar, near Aydin in Turkey). He practiced in Rome and published a 12-volume text on pathology and therapy. These volumes, translated into Latin and Arabic, were in print until the 16th century, and included a discussion on cephalalgia, cephalea, and hemicrania. He adhered to the Galenical philosophy that waste products had irritative effects upon the brain. Experiments during World War I by the Germans dispelled the common belief that toxins released in constipated individuals would cause various complaints, including headache. Soldiers were prevented from defecating for several weeks — they did not demonstrate any chemical changes within their blood measurements nor did they complain of any adverse effects with the exception of sore stomachs.

Paul of Aegina (Paulus Aegineta ca. A.D. 625 to 690) was born in Aegina (now Aiyina), one of the Dodecanese islands, and practiced in Alexandria. He described trephination — a procedure in which a circular portion of the skull bone is removed (*see color plates #1 and #2*). The ancients believed that by removing a piece of skull, the evil spirits causing the discomfort would leave through this wound. Paul gave one of the first descriptions of lead poisoning, and dealt extensively with epilepsy. He added to the list of trigger factors for migraine:

NOISES, CRIES, A BRILLIANT LIGHT, DRINKING OF WINE AND STRONG SMELLING THINGS WHICH FILL THE HEAD. SOME AS IF THE WHOLE HEAD WERE STRUCK, AND SOME AS IF ONE HALF, IN WHICH CASE THE COMPLAINT IS CALLED HEMICRANIA.

To all Christians, there were four evangelists who produced the Gospels: John, Mark, Matthew, and Luke. The first three were apostles of Jesus, but Luke was not an eye witness to the events depicted in the Gospels. Luke, a Greek-speaking native of Antioch in ancient Syria, was a disciple, friend, and "beloved physician" to St. Paul.[3] His Gospel, as well as the Acts of Apostles, were written for a gentile rather than a Jewish audience. Luke's emblem is a winged-ox, for no apparent reason (*see color plate #3*).

Diodorus, friend and employer of Aeneas, the father of Luke, was known to suffer from classic migraine (with aura). In her biography of the evangelist, *The Dear and Glorious Physician*,[4] Taylor Caldwell described the pain of Diodorus.

His headaches were often the result of scheduled confrontations with tax collectors, whom Diodorus despised. Keptah was the physician who tried to treat Diodorus, and eventually provided Luke's medical education.

❧

... HE HAD AWAKENED WITH THE DASTARDLY SUDDEN
FLASH OF LIGHT BEFORE HIS EYES, THEN THE FOLLOWING NAUSEA,
THEN THE SHARP CLEAVAGE OF VISION AND THE TEMPORARY
DIMMING OF SIGHT, AND THEN THE ACCURSED ONE-SIDED
HEADACHE. THE FACT THAT KEPTAH COULD LEARNEDLY TELL HIM IT
WAS A MIGRAINE, AND THAT HIPPOCRATES HAD WRITTEN A LONG AND
EXACT TREATISE ON IT, DID NOT ABATE ONE RETCHING, ONE HAMMER
STROKE ON THE LEFT SIDE OF HIS HEAD, OR ONE SENSATION THAT
DEATH WAS AT HAND AND NOT UNWELCOME. "MAY HADES SWALLOW
YOUR HIPPOCRATES!" HE WOULD SAY WRATHFULLY TO KEPTAH.
"NO, NO MORE OF YOUR STICKING EFFUSIONS AND THE POTIONS."
HE WOULD INVARIABLY SUBMIT TO BOTH THE EFFUSIONS AND THE
POTIONS, AND THEN WOULD TRIUMPHANTLY VOMIT BEFORE KEPTAH
AND GLARE AT HIM ACCUSINGLY. THE MIGRAINE WOULD NOT
FORSAKE HIM UNTIL EVENING.

❧

DIODORUS,
FRIEND AND EMPLOYER OF
AENEAS, THE FATHER OF LUKE,
WAS KNOWN TO SUFFER FROM
CLASSIC MIGRAINE (WITH AURA).

he most frequent ailment in the Middle East, next to dysentery, was headache (*michush rosh*).[5] Rab said, "*I can tolerate any illness but not intestinal disease, any suffering but not stomach (or heart) troubles (ke'eb leg), any pain but not headache, any evil but not an evil wife!*"[6]

The Talmud is a collection of rabbinic discussions and commentaries of biblical law. The bulk of this body of early Jewish law was created from the second through the sixth centuries.[7] The origin of headache is also speculated in the Talmud, "blowing into the foam of beverages (such as beer or mead) is damaging to the head."[8] In one episode, Rabbi Judah drank the prescribed four cups of wine on the night of Passover — the feast in which the Jews celebrate their ancient delivery from slavery in Egypt. After celebrating this holy event, Rabbi Judah was forced to bind his temples because of a severe headache.[9] Divine decree may also play a role in the occurrence of the headaches as punishment for the sins committed by the headache sufferer.

Between 20 to 40 percent of migraine sufferers believe that consumption of an alcoholic beverage will precipitate an acute attack. We do not refer to the headache caused by overconsumption but the severe attacks triggered by alcohol in susceptible individuals. Migraine patients will relate that the most frequent culprits are red wine and beer. Drinking white wines, vodka, and light scotches and whiskies does not cause the same malady. The latter drinks have a low content of agents called congeners. In small amounts, these chemicals can be tolerated by migraineurs. However, red wines, such as Chianti, have a higher tyramine count than white wines. Tyramine is known to be a substance that can cause a blood vessel to expand in those sensitive to these agents — a characteristic known to exist in migraine sufferers.

The Talmud instructs the people that in order to relieve headaches, one must occupy oneself with studying the Torah, the words of God, which *are an ornament of grace unto thy head.*[10] In one episode, the Talmud describes Jabez who prayed to God that *"thou wouldst keep from evil,"* which is interpreted to mean "that I have no headache nor earache nor eye pain."[11] The remedies for headache offered by the Talmudic sages reflect those of their Roman contemporaries, such as Celsus and Coelius Aurelianus. Headache sufferers were advised to rub the head with wine, vinegar, or oil. In its instructions for daily life, the Talmud admonishes people from visiting those suffering from headache, as speaking is harmful to them.[12] Migraine sufferers will note to their physicians that during an acute migraine attack, patients will seek the comfort of dark, quiet rooms. During the acute headache, those with migraine will relate sensitivity to light and sound. Today, migraine sufferers will often "hibernate" to a quiet, dark room to find relief of the pain and the associated symptoms.

For the majority, sleep is the best remedy for relief of their headaches. This phenomena was recognized by the ancient rabbis and their instructions hopefully aided their headaches.

Bayard Horton was a noted clinician at the Mayo Clinic in Rochester, Minnesota. His descriptions of cluster headache and the use of histamine desensitization in the treatment of headache are considered classics. Doctor Horton is considered a "headache pioneer" and was instrumental in the founding of the American Association for the Study of Headache, now the American Headache Society.

According to Doctor Horton, only one reference to headache is noted in the Bible.[13] Unfortunately, the headache has a morbid outcome:

> WHEN THE CHILD WAS OLD ENOUGH, HE WENT OUT ONE DAY
> TO THE REAPERS WHERE HIS FATHER WAS. ALL OF A SUDDEN HE
> CRIED OUT, "OH MY HEAD, MY HEAD!" HIS FATHER TOLD A SERVANT
> TO CARRY HIM TO HIS MOTHER. HE BROUGHT HIM TO HIS MOTHER;
> THE BOY SAT ON HER LAP TILL MIDDAY, THEN HE DIED. [14]

Doctor Horton suggested that the young boy had a congenital intracranial aneurysm that ruptured, causing severe, excruciating pain, and, apparently, death.

Doctor Fred Rosner, the translator of Preuss' text of medicine in the Bible and Talmud, questioned Doctor Horton's conclusion.[15] He suggested that the headache was part of the symptom complex of sunstroke, as it was the child's first exposure to the "fiercely hot Middle Eastern sun."

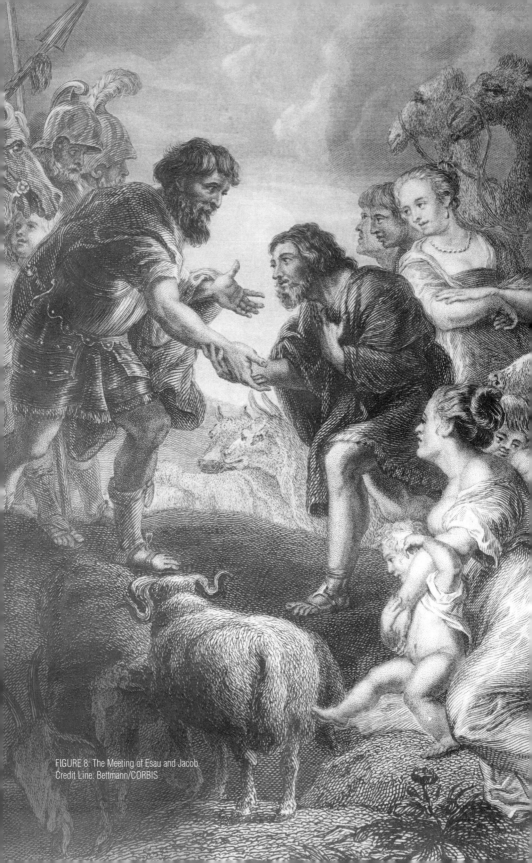

FIGURE 8: The Meeting of Esau and Jacob.
Credit Line: Bettmann/CORBIS

A.J. Bollet, the editor of *Harrison's Principles of Internal Medicine* (1984), recalled the story of Esau and Jacob, and the loss of Esau's birthright.[16] Esau, the older of the twins of Isaac and Rebekah, was an outdoors man and skilled hunter. He returned home from a prolonged hunt, weak from hunger. His twin, Jacob, offered to provide him with sustenance for the price of his birthright. Esau, feeling close to the point of dying, agreed. It is very possible that Esau was suffering from hypoglycemia, an oft-noted trigger of headache. Hypoglycemia is the state in which the blood sugar is below normal levels — an event usually produced by fasting or missing a meal. As a general measure to reduce headaches, physicians treating headache patients will advise them to maintain regular meal schedules and avoid missing a meal.

AS A GENERAL MEASURE TO REDUCE HEADACHES, PHYSICIANS TREATING HEADACHE PATIENTS WILL ADVISE THEM TO MAINTAIN REGULAR MEAL SCHEDULES AND AVOID MISSING A MEAL.

HEADACHE IN THE MIDDLE AGES

After the dissolution of the Roman Empire, Greek medical traditions did not disappear but were maintained in the universities of the Arab world. Fortunately for all of us, the ancient manuscripts were preserved at the Arabic centers of learning, and incorporated into the curriculum of medical students. The Arab surgeons utilized the Greek and Roman texts, such as Galen's, for their anatomical descriptions. The Near East was abundant with plants from which drugs could be extracted — a practice well documented by the Arab physicians. In approximately A.D. 754, the first apothecary shop was established in Baghdad in ancient Iraq. This occurrence marked the first known division of the professions of pharmacy and medicine.

The most important physician in this world was Avicenna (A.D. 980 to 1037). His contributions to science and philosophy are incredible. His *Canons of Medicine*, a systematic exposition of the accomplishments of the Greek and Roman physicians, became the definitive work in the medical field for many centuries but unfortunately provides meager discussion on headache. He was born in Bukhara, Persia (now Iran), and by the age of 21, was

ISLAMIC SPAIN

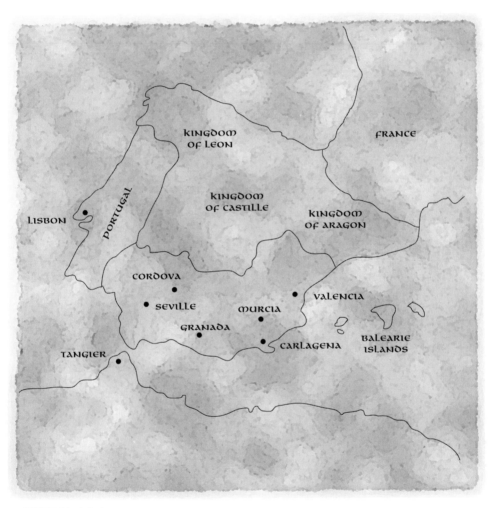

FIGURE 9: Islamic Spain

known as an outstanding scholar and physician. He traveled throughout Persia, and completed *The Book of Healing,* which was a large encyclopedia covering the natural sciences, logic, mathematics, psychology, astronomy, music, and philosophy. This project is one of the most extensive endeavors completed by one scholar. His career, however, was cut short by alcoholism. During the century following his death, his work was translated into Latin, affording its availability to the scientists of Europe.

Avicenna called headache *soda,* from the Persian word *sar did.* He observed that headache location could be frontal, occipital (at the back of the head), or generalized. If the headache was typically one sided, it was termed hemicrania. Avicenna noted that smells could provoke soda in normal people. He also observed that cashews, used for practically all psychiatric and neural afflictions, were appropriate headache remedies. During Avicenna's time, the Arab physicians also utilized *anomum nelegueta,* an African ginger, for headache, epilepsy, and syncope.

During the Umayyad caliphate, Cordoba, the capital and cultural center of Islamic Spain, also flourished in the pursuit of scientific knowledge. Abã al-Q~sim (Abulcasis) was the royal physician to the Spanish caliph, and considered the greatest of Islam's medieval surgeons. Abulcasis wrote the first illustrated text on surgery, *at-Tasr§f,* which was the leading surgical textbook in Europe for the next 500 years. One recommendation for headache treatment was noninvasive, however anything but conservative. Abulcasis suggested that a hot iron should be applied to the head of the sufferer, perhaps in an effort to forget their presenting symptom. But true to his surgeon's identity, Abulcasis also suggested making an incision in the temple and applying garlic to the site.

Cordoba was also the birthplace of the most prominent scholar of medieval Judaism, Maimonides (1135 to 1204). Moses ben Maimon, also known as Rambam, was a prolific writer in philosophy, religion, and medicine. His family fled to Fez, Morocco, to escape persecution from a fanatical Islamic sect. There, Maimonides began his medical studies, only to again flee, this time to Palestine and then to Egypt. His reputation as a physician attracted the notice of the Visier Al-Fadhil, the Regent of Egypt, during the absence of the Sultan, Saladin, who was off fighting the European crusaders. Legend has it that Maimonides was visited by Richard the Lion-Hearted, King of England, who asked Maimonides to serve as his physician — an offer he refused.[17] In addition to his works on the philosophy of Judaism and his code of Jewish law which are legendary, Maimonides also contributed heavily to the study of medicine — works that are still studied.

Maimonides was heavily influenced by Galen and Hippocrates, as illustrated by his description of headache:

❧

THICK VISCOUS HUMORS CAUSE HEADACHE. ALL THICK BLACK HUMORS [IE, BLACK BILE] CAUSE HEADACHES IF THEY ARE RETAINED IN THE PASSAGES OF THE CAVITIES OF THE BRAIN IF THIS [BLACK HUMOR] PREVAILS AND INCREASES IN THE BRAIN SUBSTANCE ITSELF, BLACK CONFUSION [MELANCHOLY OR DEPRESSION] ENSUES.[17]

❧

Maimonides also commented on other triggers of headache:

❧

"SEVERE HEADACHE OCCURS FROM HEAT OR COLD. ON THE OTHER HAND, HEADACHE PRODUCED BY DRYNESS IS MILD WHEREAS MOISTURE CAUSES NO [HEAD] PAIN AT ALL. HOWEVER, IF MUCH MOISTURE IS PRESENT IN THE HEAD, A HEAVINESS IS PRODUCED, NOT [TRUE] PAIN, UNLESS THE ILLNESS CALLED VERTIGO, OTHERWISE KNOWN AS SCOTODINIA, ENSUES THEREFROM. HEADACHE OCCURS PROPORTIONAL TO THE DEGREE OF OBSTRUCTION."

❧

Decreases in barometric pressure have been identified as migraine triggers. Some patients will complain of headaches related to changes in weather. Triggers include cold weather; hot, dry winds such as the sirocco of the Sahara; the onset of humid, hot weather; or rapidly falling atmospheric pressure. Migraine patients will describe an increase in attacks related to high-altitude flights or mountain vacations — both scenarios due to diminished barometric pressure.

In his writings, Maimonides also notes some treatments:

PEOPLE WHO SUFFER FROM A STRONG MIDLINE HEADACHE
[IE MIGRAINE] OR THE LIKE SECONDARY TO THICK BLOOD OR
INTERNAL COLDNESS ARE OVERTLY BENEFITTED BY DRINKING
UNDILUTED WINE EITHER AFTER A MEAL OR DURING THE MEAL.
THEIR PAIN IS ALLEVIATED BY THE WARMING EFFECT OF THE WINE
AND ITS THINNING [OF THE BLOOD]. ALSO, FEED THEM BREAD OR
TOAST [SOAKED] IN UNDILUTED WINE BECAUSE THE MIXING OF PURE
WINE WITH FOOD WILL POSITIVELY PREVENT THE ASCENT OF WARM
GASES FROM IT WHICH ARE HARMFUL AT THE SITE OF THE PAIN.

He recommended that headache sufferers should refrain
from physical exertion and other activities until the pain begins
to diminish — a thought shared by many afflicted by headache.
Maimonides warned the headache sufferers to avoid eating fruit
rich in moisture, such as melons, peaches, apricots, mulberries,
fresh dates, etc.[18]

Maimonides did not believe that medication should be
taken for a mild headache — nature could relieve without assis-
tance. Conducting a normal healthy life was sufficient to avoid
headaches. In his legal code, Maimonides notes that a man with
headache is considered legally as in good health in regard to the
validity of his buying, selling, and giving of gifts.[19, 20]

FOR HEADACHES, FRANKISH KINGS UNDERWENT SURGERY UNDER THE WATCHFUL EYE OF THEIR WARRIORS.

Medical historians have access to documents relating to headache therapies of Islamic Spain, but very little is available from medieval Christian Europe. As early as sixth century France, we can encounter a discourse on headache treatment. The author, St. Gregory, Bishop of Tours, was an early travel agent, promoting the importance of pilgrimages to shrines recognized in his early Christian world. His own experience of a cure for a headache was attributed to pressing his head to the altar rail surrounding the sepulcher (a place for internment of a dead body) of the tomb of St. Martin of Tours. St. Gregory also recommended a relief from headaches by touching the carpet over the resting place of St. Julian. For headaches, Frankish kings underwent surgery under the watchful eye of their warriors.

During this period, medical treatment was often limited to the monastic life. The Irish monks were travelers throughout western Europe, establishing monasteries along the way. A hymn from the 8th century was found among the manuscripts stored at the Monastery of Reichenau at Lake Constance. As translated, the prayer follows:

O King, o ruler of the realm,
o friend of heaven's hymn,
o persecutor of turmoil,
o God of the heavenly Host!
Aed o goodwilled St. Mac Bricc.
From the pure I ask the prayers
That he cools the noxious fluxes
That flow heated in my head,
That he cures my head with my kidneys,
And with the other parts afflicted:
With my eyes and with my cheekbones.
With my ears and with my nostrils.
With the famous emanations,
And with the resounding conduits.
With the tongue and with the teeth,
And the fountains of the tears.
Holy Aed on high does help me
That he does my head deliver,
That he keps it all in good health,
That he keeps it all protected.

The St. Aed has been identified as Aed Mac Bricc, a 6th century Irish bishop, who was known for miracles of healing and extraordinary astuteness. In one story, translated from Colgan's *Acta Sanctorum Hiberniae*[21]:

A MAN WHO WAS SUFFERING FROM A GREAT PAIN IN THE
HEAD CAME TO ST. AED AND SAID: O HOLY MAN OF GOD
I AM VERY PLAGUED BY HEADACHE, AND PRAY FOR ME.
THE BISHOP SAID TO HIM: IN NO WAY WILL THAT PAIN
DEPART FROM YOU, UNLESS IT WILL COME OVER ME:
BUT YOU WILL GAIN GREAT MERIT, IF YOU BEAR IT PATIENTLY.
HE ANSWERED: SIR, THE PAIN IS BEYOND MY FORCES. ST. AED SAID:
THE PAIN IN YOUR HEAD, O MAN, MAY COME INTO
MY HEAD. AND IMMEDIATELY THE PAIN DESCENDED INTO THE
BISHOP'S HEAD, AND THAT MAN WENT OUT HEALTHY
AND GIVING THANKS.

The early Irish Christians would invoke the name of St. Aed to relieve them of head pain. Legend has it that St. Bridget prayed to St. Aed and her headaches disappeared.

Illuminated manuscripts originally started in Egyptian times with the *Book of the Dead*. The Greeks and Romans illustrated mathematical, medical, and other scientific and literary texts. The tradition of medieval manuscript illumination is overwhelmingly religious and moralizing *(see color plate #3)*.

In an 8th century Irish manuscript, an incantation was provided that promised relief from pain in the head. The reader was advised to intone a prayer to "the eye of Isaia, the tongue of Solomon, the mind of Benjamin, the heart of St. Paul and the faith of Abraham." The prayer was to end with *"Sanctus, sanctus, Dominus, Deus, Sabaoth."* To be successful, the incantation was to be repeated each day, followed by "placing the spittle upon thy palm and putting it on thy temples and at the back of thy head and reciting the Pater (the Our Father) thrice thereupon and draw a cross with thy spittle on the top of thy head and on thy head also draw the form of the letter U."[22]

The next century in the British Isles did not find any startling cure. In one manuscript, the headache sufferer was encouraged to apply to the forehead, a concoction made from swallows' nest and boiled in water. In a medieval prescription, the patient is to "Take the juice of elderseed, cow's brain, and goat's dung dissolved in vinegar."[23] Hopefully, the headache sufferer used it as a poultice and not an oral analgesic. The elder seed probably referred to the European alder, *Alnus vulgaris.*

The curative powers of the willow bark was also noted at this time. Herbalists recommended its use for all types of painful conditions. However, its popularity was curtailed as the immediate need for the stalks in basket weaving outweighed its usefulness in pain management.

In the 12th century, a woman of extraordinary intelligence and talent emerged as a leader in her own Benedictine community and within the Church. Hildegard, Abbess of Bingen (1098 to 1179), in the Rhine valley of Germany, was renowned for her oratory abilities in her preaching, for her talent in composing religious music, and for authoring texts on a multitude of subjects. She was an extraordinary organizer and reformer in an age when the opinions of women were, at best, ignored. She traveled throughout western Europe, and was known to admonish anyone of whom she disapproved, including the Holy Roman Emperor, Frederick Barbarossa. Her religious music, including 72 songs, is still studied, particularly by feminist scholars. Her books include one on physiology, *Liber Simplicis Medicinae*, and a treatise on botany and biology, with pharmaceutical advise, *Physica*.

However, we will focus on her illuminated manuscripts, in which Hildegard depicted her spiritual visions, images that she believed were divinely inspired. It is now accepted that the Abbess was experiencing the symptoms of migraine aura. She may have seen the jagged lines and bright lights associated with the aura *(see color plate #5).*

Hildegard's canonization has been attempted on three occasions, the last under Pope John XXII in 1317. Some recognize her sainthood based on her inclusion in the list of

Roman martyrs who were automatically named saints in the 12th century. Her cult, within and without the Church, has continued, and in 1979, Pope John Paul II, on the 800th anniversary of Hildegard's death, remarked that she was "an outstanding saint a light to her people and her time (who) shines out more brightly today."[24]

About the time of Hildegard's visions, on the other side of the Rhine, the populace was afflicted with an outbreak of ergotism or St. Anthony's fire, due to spoiled rye. Ergotism is manifested by the death of the tissue in the extremities. These symptoms results from contraction of the blood vessels in the legs and arms. It is presumed that on the Bingen side of the mighty river, the spoiled crop led to an increase in migraine symptoms in afflicted individuals. Hildegard, along with some of her neighbors, experienced visions during this time. Some of the visions could be due to the mental effects of the ergot poisoning. Hallucinations are common in ergot-exposed individuals.

Hildegard described her first vision as:

"TO COME TO LIGHT IN THE KNOWLEDGE OF MYSTERIES . . . WHERE
WITH A BRIGHT LIGHT THIS SERENITY WILL SHINE FORTH STRONGLY
AMONG THOSE WHO SHINE FORTH."[24]

We have come to use her visual imagery as excellent examples of the visual symptoms of the aura:

❧

"I SAW A GREAT STAR MOST SPLENDID AND BEAUTIFUL,
AND WITH IT AN EXCEEDING MULTITUDE OF FALLING SPARKS WHICH
WITH THE STAR FOLLOWED SOUTHWARD . . . AND SUDDENLY THEY
WERE ALL ANNIHILATED, BEING TURNED INTO BLACK COALS. . . .
THE LIGHT WHICH I SEE IS NOT LOCATED BUT YET IS MORE BRILLIANT
THAN THE SUN, NOR CAN I EXAMINE ITS HEIGHT, LENGTH,
OR BREADTH, AND I NAME IT 'THE CLOUD OF THE LIVING LIGHT . . .'
BUT SOMETIMES I BEHOLD WITHIN THIS LIGHT ANOTHER LIGHT . . .
ALL THESE I SEE NOT WITH THE OUTWARD EYE . . .
BUT WITHIN MY SPIRIT, MY EYES BEING OPEN."[25]

❧

In Hildegard's view, there is no distinction between physical events, moral truths, and spiritual experiences.[25] She described periodic attacks of a vague nature, with complete recovery between attacks (*see color plate #6*). However, there is no evidence that after experiencing the visions did she suffer from any type of headache. She noted that after her visions, "I have never suffered any terror when they left me." It would not be unusual for the prodromal symptoms to occur without a resulting headache.[26] We can appreciate the legacy left by Hildegard and her illuminations, for they vividly depict the visual symptoms of the migraine aura. In one vision, "The Fall of Angels," she has brilliantly rendered a scintillating scotoma:[27]

> "I SAW A GREAT STAR MOST SPLENDID AND BEAUTIFUL,
> AND WITH IT AN EXCEEDING MULTITUDE OF FALLING SPARKS
> WHICH THE STAR FOLLOWED SOUTHWARD. AND THEY
> EXAMINED HIM UPON HIS THRONE."

It should be noted that many migraine sufferers will note a decrease and possibly a complete remission of the attacks as they advance in age. For those with migraine with aura, another type of attack may occur. For some individuals, the headache pain will cease but they will experience episodes of the aura — without a succeeding headache. Many of these individuals will consult a variety of medical specialists, including ophthalmologists, due to fears that they are suffering from a serious neurological disorder, such as a brain tumor or aneurysm. In reality, they are experiencing a silent manifestation of their migraine attacks.

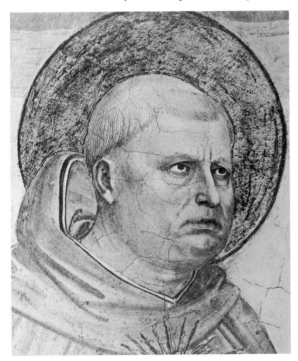

FIGURE 10: Saint Thomas Aquinas (1225?–1274)
An Italian scholastic philosopher is depicted here.
The detail is from "Fresco" by Fra Angelico.
(Florence S. Marco Museum)
Credit Line: Bettmann/CORBIS

During the next century, the treatment of headache in the Christian world continued to look to mystical cures.[28] St. Albert the Great (Albert Magnus) (1193? to 1280), was born in Swabia, Germany. He was a scholar, scientist, and Doctor of the Church, as well as the teacher of St. Thomas Aquinas. He recommended using "arnoglasse," a plant under the dominion of the planet Mars.[26] In addition to his theological expertise, St. Albert utilized astrology for some of his theories. Mars was synonymous with the zodiac sign, Aries, which was believed to predispose its subjects to headaches. The name "arnoglosse" does not appear in botanical nomenclature, and was probably coined by the saint himself. *Glossa*, in Greek, refers to the tongue and could have referred to a projecting portion of the plant. *Arn* is an old Scottish word for the alder tree, which was previously recommended as a headache treatment. St. Albert would be welcomed by the conservative right today, as he maintained that frequent intercourse could lead to sickness, body odor, baldness, and could cause one's brain to shrink to the size of a pomegranate. He was not canonized until 700 years after his death, in 1941, when he was declared by Pope Pius XII to be the Patron of Scientists.

His famous student, Thomas Aquinas (1224 to 1274), was born Thomas d'Aquino, in Roccasecca, Italy. He is regarded as the Catholic Church's greatest theologian and philosopher. St. Albert introduced Thomas to the works of Aristotle, and the student endeavored to incorporate the teachings of the Greek philosopher into Christian doctrine. The Patron of Scholars, Theologians, and Pencil Makers, and the author of *Summa Contra Gentiles* and *Summa Theologiae*, Thomas is often listed as one of the many famous migraine sufferers. He is of peculiar importance in the Middle Ages because of his carefulness, subtlety, and precision with which he handled questions about philosophy and theology. These features of carefulness and precision have often been identified with the so-called migraine personality.

Many studies have emerged on the psychological patterns of migraine sufferers. The role of suppressed anger has long been identified.[29] Studies during the 1940s revealed patients with migraine had a tendency toward rigidity, persistence toward success, difficulty in sexual adjustment, perfectionism, conventionality, intolerance, and obsessive-compulsive features.[30] These data were refuted by reports during the 1980s.[31] In one of the author's clinical experience, he has observed the traits of perfectionism, compulsiveness, and rigidity occurring commonly in migraine sufferers. Throughout history, those figures identified as headache sufferers often "fit" this personality type.

Throughout the 13th and 14th centuries, herbal medicine was the recognized remedy for headache. Magical properties were attributed to several species of the genus of herbs, *Artemisia*. Some scholars felt that the ancient Greeks originated this belief, denoting a relationship with the moon goddess, Artemis. These herbs were considered quite beneficial during the late Middle Ages. *A. Vulgaris* (mugwort) and *A. Absinthium* (wormwood) were frequently cited in the literature. In one formula from Bohemia, the headache sufferer was advised to weave one of the herbs into a garland and wear it on the hair or view the customary midsummer bonfire through it, in order to relieve headaches and eye problems for the upcoming year. Bartholomew of England, a contemporary of Thomas Aquinas, compiled an extensive summary of current human knowledge, *De Proprietatibus Rerum* (On the Properties of Things). In the 7th volume of this work, Bartholomew discussed medical topics. For headache treatment, he recommended a cure, believed to evolve from the time of Emperor Constantine, to scarify the shinbones. Scarification involves making a number of cuts, scratches, incisions, or scars on the skin or the mucous membrane. The theory behind this remedy was to transfer the injurious humor from the head to the lower extremities.

HEADACHE IN THE RENAISSANCE

MY HEED DID ACHE SO YESTERNIGCHT.
THIS DAY TAE MAK THAT I NAY MIGCHT.
SO SPIR THE MYGRINE DOES MY MENEYE.
PERSING MY BROW AS ONY GANEYE THAT
SCANT I LUIK MAY ON THE LIGCHT.

— *William Dunbar, 15th century Scottish poet*

illiam Dunbar (1460 to 1521) was a poet of the late Middle Ages. Intending to have most of his poetry read at court, he wrote in the Middle Scots language, which is considered a high point in Scottish literature — and making its reading difficult for those in the 21st century. Like his contemporaries, Dunbar focused on allegories, using elaborate diction. He also wrote on ordinary life, such as the above description of a headache.

By the Renaissance, Galen's teachings were losing ground in European medicine, and the physicians began to

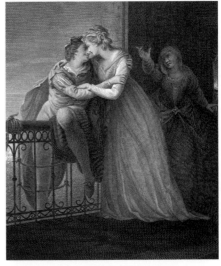

FIGURE 11: *Romeo Takes Leave of Juliet* by James Stow
A print showing Act 3, Scene 5 from *Romeo and Juliet* by William Shakespeare. This engraving is based after a painting by John Francis Rigaud. Date created: 1797
Credit Line: Bettmann/CORBIS

seek a scientific basis for their treatments and diagnoses. New principles of anatomy were discovered through the systematic dissection of human bodies. Old habits die hard, as barbers were still considered surgeons, combining hair cutting with minor surgical procedures, trauma care, and bloodletting. Barbers, however, were not considered sufficiently respectable to be physicians. Bloodletting, developed by physicians, was believed to have a curative effect on disease, although it hastened the death of many patients. It was not abandoned as a common medical intervention until the 18th century.

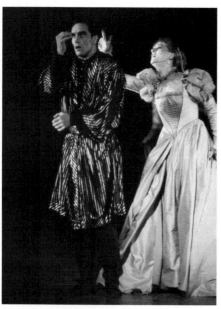

FIGURE 12: Irek Mukhamedov and Leesa Phillips in *Othello*.
Date photographed: February 1994
Credit Line: Robbie Jack/CORBIS

The bane of headache found its way into the plays of Shakespeare.[32] Juliet's nurse in *Romeo and Juliet*, Act II, suffered a headache, probably a migraine, on the eve of her mistress' wedding: "Lord, how my head aches! What a head have I! It beats as it would fall in twenty pieces." The doomed Desdemona, in Othello, Act III, displays her empathy with her pained husband in the following dialogue:

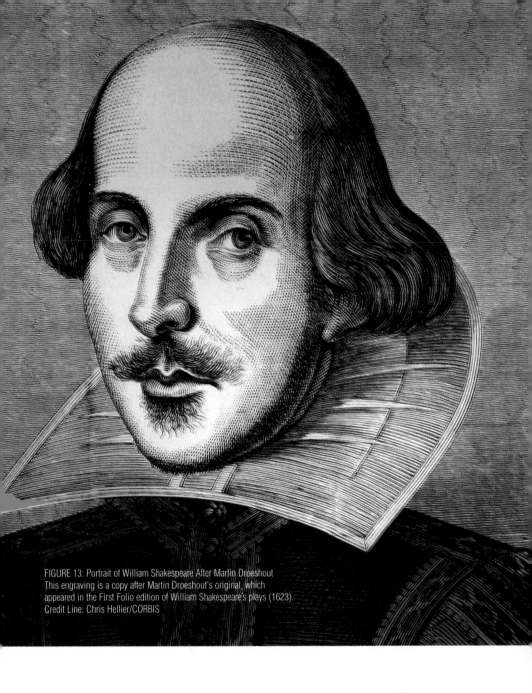

FIGURE 13: Portrait of William Shakespeare After Martin Droeshout
This engraving is a copy after Martin Droeshout's original, which
appeared in the First Folio edition of William Shakespeare's plays (1623).
Credit Line: Chris Hellier/CORBIS

Desdemona: *Why do you speak so faintly? Are you not well?*

Othello: *I have a pain upon my forehead here.*

Desdemona: *Let me but bind it hard, within this hour — It will be well.*

The tight band which we first saw in the Talmud makes another appearance. It most probably alludes to the occurrence of tension-type headaches which are usually described as caplike, vise-like, and tight headband sensations around the head. Unlike migraine, tension-type headaches are not one-sided. The pain can radiate to the neck or shoulders. Other descriptions of this form of headache include pressure, cramplike, weight, and fullness. Patients may complain of pain when combing or brushing the hair or when putting on a hat.

Headache also found its way into the halls of royalty. Mary, Queen of Scotland (1542 to 1587), a noted migraineur, lost her head, literally, due to her cousin, Elizabeth I, of England. She inherited the throne of Scotland a few days after her birth when her father, King James V of Scotland, died. Her mother, the French princess Mary of Guise, sent the child to France to be trained in the graces of court life. The child queen had originally been betrothed to Prince Edward of England but the Scots, fearing that Edward's father, Henry VIII, would annex Scotland to England, betrothed Mary to the Dauphin Francis of France. In 1558, when Mary finally married the Dauphin, her cousin Elizabeth became Queen of England — succeeding her father, Henry VIII, her brother Edward, and her sister Mary Tudor. In 1560, the king of France died, and Queen Mary returned to Scotland to rule. The Protestant reformation had reached Scotland, and as a Catholic monarch, Mary was denounced from the pulpit and feared by her Protestant cousin in England. If Elizabeth should die childless, Catholic cousin Mary was the next heir to the English throne — a prospect especially distasteful to Queen Elizabeth and her court. After many machinations and treachery, Mary was arrested and forced to abdicate to her infant son, James VI, the son of her second husband, Lord Darnley, who had been assassinated.

In her biography, the following details her coronation procession:

"... MARY RODE IN AN OPEN LITTER, CLAD IN SPLENDID BLUE VELVET,
WITH A JEWELED DIADEM SO HEAVY THAT ITS WEIGHT ON
THE USUAL HEADACHE — SHE WAS HAVING ONE OF HER BAD DAYS —
WAS SHEER AGONY, SO THAT FOR PART OF THE WAY SHE TRIED
TO EASE THE BLIND PAIN BY RESTING HER HEAD ON HER HAND."[22]

Another famous Renaissance figure, known to have suffered migraine, was the great reformer, John Calvin (1509 to 1564). During Calvin's childhood in France, Martin Luther launched the Protestant Reformation in Germany. Calvin had studied in Paris for the priesthood and became unsettled when learning of Luther's ideas, eventually leaving the Catholic church. His *Institutes of the Christian Religion*, published in 1536, became a rallying point for Protestants throughout Europe. Forced to flee France, Calvin moved to Geneva, Switzerland, and rose to be a powerful figure in the social and cultural life of this "city of God." Calvin forced his ideas on purity, simplicity, and devout religious faith on the city, and Geneva became one of the most influential cities in Europe. The teachings of Calvin are the basis of the Presbyterian and Reformed churches, spreading to France, the Netherlands, Scotland, England, and eventually to the New World with the Pilgrims of Massachusetts.

Physicians of the time were contributing to the thoughts on migraine. Charles Lepois (Carolus Piso) (1563 to 1633), completed a monograph, *Hemicrania*. This treatise focuses primarily on the author's headache attacks which started during his days as a student. The headaches were only relieved by sleep or vomiting (an acknowledged feature of migraine) or by the consumption of excessive amounts of fluid. Lepois' headaches were influenced by weather changes. He described the pain as if the head were splitting in two. In describing the sleepiness or stupor produced by the headache, Galen's influence on his thoughts is evident: *"A not unwelcome bewitching or drugging of the pain"* — and was attributed to the differential effect of the four humors upon the brain. Lepois also considered one-sided headache as related to epilepsy.

John Churchill, the first Duke of Marlborough and ancestor of Winston Churchill, is a famed headache sufferer of this time. His military achievements and opportune desertion of the army of James II of England to the new king, William of Orange, gained him the title of Duke and commander-in-chief of the British forces. His successes in the Battle of the Spanish Succession helped thwart France from gaining control of Spain and its many colonies. As a reward, Blenheim Palace was built for him, a site that would later gain fame as the birthplace of Winston Churchill, the great World War II prime minister *(see color plate #7)*.

HEADACHE IN THE 17TH CENTURY

The 17th century saw a new age of medicine. Nicholas Culpeper (1616 to 1654) established himself as an herbalist-physician-astrologer in London. In 1649, Culpeper published the English translation of the *Pharmacopoeia*, which was upsetting to his colleagues who kept their medical formulae secret by publishing in Latin. For nervous headache, Culpeper prescribed valerian, also known as the "phew plant" because of its offensive odor. Valerian is a perennial herb that was used as a carminative (remedy for colic or flatulence) and as a sedative, especially in nervous conditions. The use of valerian for headaches continued into the 19th century. Its sedative actions appear to explain its success in combating nervous tension.

Roses and candied sugar were also accepted as headache remedies during the 17th century. In a recipe dated from 1657, a piece of "A Red Rose Cake, moistened therewith with vinegar of roses, should be cut first for the head and heated between a double-folded cloth, with a little beaten nutmeg and poppy seed, strewed on the side that must lie next to the forehead and temples and bound so thereto for all night."[33] During this time, both Christians and Jews relied on the efficacy of the magical rituals, such as incantations, prayers, inscriptions, holy water, and similar

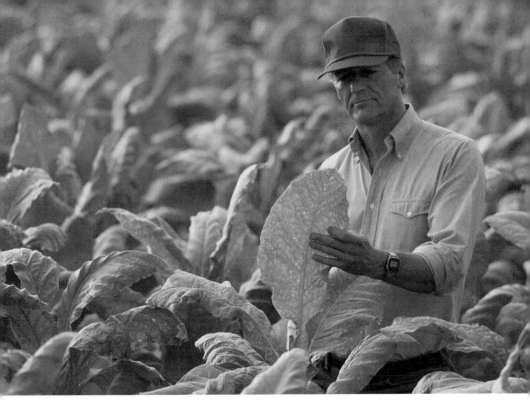

FIGURE 14: Farmer Inspecting Tobacco, Credit Line: Chuck Savage/CORBIS

efforts to exorcise pain-causing demons from "possessed" individuals. In one French account, a young French nun, in 1613, was believed to be possessed by several devils, each holding sway over a portion of her head, and she was cured by intensive exorcism during a period of 4 months.[34]

In Italy, a professor at the University of Bologna, recommended a solution of geraniums, *G. Maculatum*, to be placed on the head. Atropa belladonna was first recommended during this time but was not used internally. Its leaves were applied to the head to relieve headache and insomnia.[35]

When the explorers arrived in the New World during the 16th and 17th centuries, they found that headache was not segregated to Europe. The Indians of North and South America had been using *Nicotiana tabacum*, tobacco, as snuff, and used it for headaches, labor pains, and asthma. The Indians also used the testes of the beaver bottled in spirits as a remedy for nervous headaches. This prescription was not accepted in Europe, which may have delayed an important find in headache medicine. The secretion from the beaver contained a salicylate-like agent, perhaps derived from the bark of trees that beavers typically consume.

The contributions of Thomas Willis to the 17th century knowledge of headache are immeasurable. He was born in Wiltshire, England, in 1621, and died in London in 1675. Willis is interred at Westminster Abbey. Willis served with Royalist troops during the English Civil War, and he was independent from traditional Galenic and Aristotelian beliefs which were then taught at Oxford.[36] Because he was not in step with the Puritan leadership, Willis was one of the founders of the Royal Society, with other supporters of the "New" or experimental science. He practiced in Oxford and London, and was considered the leader of the iatrochemical school in England.

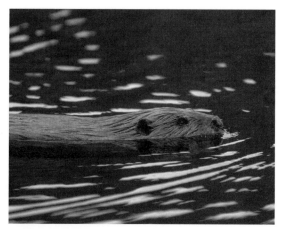

FIGURE 15: Beaver Swimming in Pond. ca. 1992
Denali National Park and Reserve, Alaska, USA
Credit Line: Charles Mauzy/CORBIS

Iatrochemistry refers to the combination of medicine and chemistry. It was used during the period of 1525 to 1660. Willis was also considered an exceptional clinician, and is best remembered for his description of the *Cerebri anatome*, the ring of communicating vessels under the base of the brain — better known as the Circle of Willis.

As other physicians of his time, he sought a cure to replace the many ineffective therapies then available:

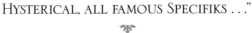

"FOR THE OBTAINING A CUR; OR RATHER FOR A TRYAL
VERY MANY REMEDIES WERE ADMINISTERED, THOROW THE
WHOLE PROGRESS OF THE DISEASE, BY THE MOST SKILFUL
PHYSICIANS . . . WITHOUT ANY SUCCESS OR EASE . . .
AN OINTMENT OF QUICKSILVER . . . A FLUX AT THE MOUTH FROM A
MERCURIAL POWDER . . . BATH, AND THE SPAWWATERS
ALMOST OF EVERY KIND AND NATURE; THERE WAS NO KIND
OF MEDICINE BOTH CEPHALICKS, ANTISCROBUTTICKS,
HYSTERICAL, ALL FAMOUS SPECIFIKS . . ."

His care of Ann Finch, who later became the Lady Conway, was a great opportunity to observe a patient from age 12 to her death at 48.[37] Her headaches were violent and periodic, and she described the pain and the associated exhaustion to her husband, the Earl of Conway:

"I CANNOT DISSEMBLE SO MUCH AS TO PROFESS
MYSELF VERY WEARY OF THIS CONDITION."

His case study on Lady Conway is one of the most illustrative of the various symptoms of migraine.

Willis also provided an excellent description of premonitory symptoms before a headache. Patients may describe vague symptoms occurring as early as 48 hours prior to the acute headache. Fatigue, bursts of energy, and hunger are included in these premonitory symptoms:

"... BEAUTIFUL AND YOUNG WOMAN, INDUED WITH A SLENDER HABIT OF BODY, AND AN HOT BLOOD, BEING OBNOXIOUS TO AN HEREDITARY HEADACH, WAS WONT TO BE AFFLICTED WITH FREQUENT AND WANDERING FITS OF IT, TO WIT, SOME UPON EVERY LIGHT OCCASION, AND SOME OF THEIR OWN ACCORD; THAT IS ARISING, WITHOUT ANY EVIDENT CAUSE. ON THE DAY BEFORE THE COMING OF THE SPONTANEOUS FIT OF THIS DISEASE, GROWING VERY HUNGRY IN THE EVENING, SHE EAT A MOST PLENTIFUL SUPPER, WITH AN HUNGRY, I MAY SAY A GREEDY APPETITE; PRESAGING BY THIS SIGN, THAT THE PAIN OF THE HEAD WOULD MOST CERTAINLY FOLLOW THE NEXT MORNING; AND THE EVENT NEVER FALED THIS AUGURY. FOR AS SOON AS SHE AWAKED, BEING AFFLICTED BY A MOST SHARP TORMENT, THOROW THE WHOLEFOREPART OF HER HEAD, SHE WAS TROUBLED ALSO WITH VOMITING, SOMETIMES OF AN ACID, AND AS IT WERE A BITRIOLOCK, HUMOR, AND SOMETIMES OF A CHOLERICK AND HIGHLY BITTERISH; HENCE ACCORDING TO THIS SIGN THIS HEADACH IS THOUGHT TO ARISE FROM THE VICE OF THE STOMACH."

Miguel de Cervantes Saavedra (1547 to 1616), was a Spanish novelist, dramatist, and poet. He originally served in the military, but lost the use of his left hand in the Battle of Lepanto (1571), and tenure as a prisoner in Algiers (1575 to 1580) caused a career change to civil servant. Late in his life, he was able to obtain a patron and give full attention to his writing.

❧

WHEN THE HEAD ACHES, ALL THE MEMBERS
PARTAKE OF THE PAINS.[38]

❧

— *Don Quixote*

Cervantes is best known for his classic novel, *Don Quixote de la Mancha*, the saga of a knight-errant who behaves according to

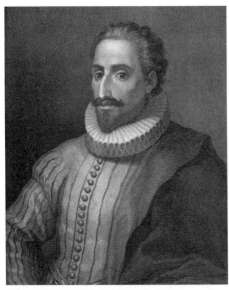

a code of chivalry from a bygone age. Most critics believe that despite the humorous content of Don Quixote's misadventures, his purpose in the novel is to examine the value of idealism. In his quest, Cervantes also contributed to the headache literature. A pain in the head can affect the entire body, whether with generalized pain or accompanying nausea and vomiting.

FIGURE 16: Portrait of Miguel de Cervantes Saavedra (1547–1616), Spanish author whose novel *Don Quixote* (1605) made him the most celebrated figure in Spanish literature.
Date Created: 1791
Credit Line: Bettmann/CORBIS

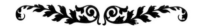

HEADACHE TYPES AND NOTABLE PEOPLE AFFECTED BY THEM THROUGH THE 20TH CENTURY

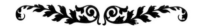

THE MAJORITY OF THE HEADACHES SEEN BY A GENERALIST WILL BE OF A TRANSIENT NATURE, AND WILL BE OF MINOR, NONPERMANENT CONSEQUENCE TO THE PATIENT. THESE HEADACHES OFTEN ARE EPISODIC IN THEIR OCCURRENCE AND ARE BEST MANAGED WITH OVER-THE-COUNTER NONSTEROIDAL ANTI-INFLAMMATORY AGENTS, SUCH AS ASPIRIN, IBUPROFEN, ACETAMINOPHEN, KETOPROFEN, OR NAPROXEN SODIUM. HOWEVER, FOR MANY INDIVIDUALS, THE BANE OF HEADACHE IS A CHRONIC, DEBILITATING, PAIN CONDITION WHICH CAN GREATLY IMPACT ON FAMILY AND SOCIAL LIFE, AND BE A TREMENDOUS FINANCIAL BURDEN. IN THE PREVIOUS CHAPTER, WE HAVE SEEN HEADACHE FROM A HISTORICAL PERSPECTIVE. ANCIENT WRITERS HAVE DEPICTED THIS MALADY IN LITERATURE AND PAINTINGS. WE WILL NOW FOCUS ON THREE FORMS OF HEADACHES THAT USUALLY REQUIRE MEDICAL INTERVENTION, ALTHOUGH THEY ARE NOT LIFE-THREATEN-ING — MIGRAINE, CLUSTER, AND CHRONIC TENSION-TYPE.

IN ORDER TO UNDERSTAND THE HEADACHE PROBLEMS AND APPROPRIATELY MANAGE THESE ATTACKS, THE PHYSICIAN MUST APPRE-CIATE WHY THE PAIN IS THERE. ONE MUST REALIZE THAT HEADACHE IS A SYMPTOM AND NOT A SOLITARY DISEASE. PAIN ITSELF IS A SUBJECTIVE COMPLAINT, RENDERING IN MANY CASES, DEFINITIVE TESTING OF THE DEGREE AND QUALITY OF THE PAIN IMPOSSIBLE.

ONE MUST REALIZE THAT HEADACHE IS A SYMPTOM AND NOT A SOLITARY DISEASE.

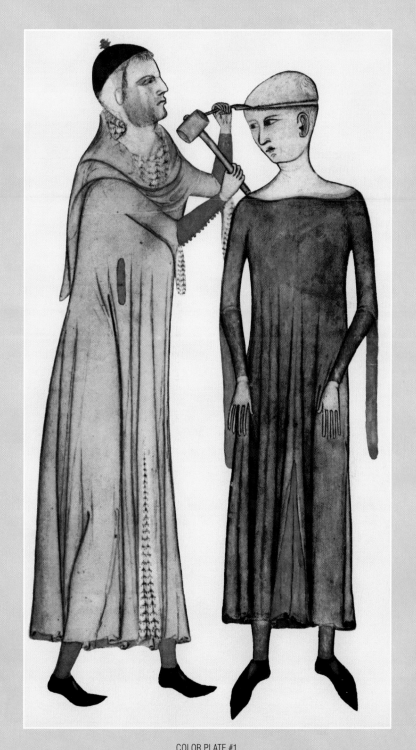

COLOR PLATE #1
Murphy W, and the editors of Time-Life Books. *Dealing With Headaches.* Chicago, Ill: Time-Life Books Inc.; 1982:25.
Using a mallet and trepan, a medieval surgeon chisels a hole in his patient's skull, in an illustration from a 14th Century Italian anatomical treatise.
One contemporary medical textbook cautioned: "If it is necessary to strike with the mallet let this be done gently."

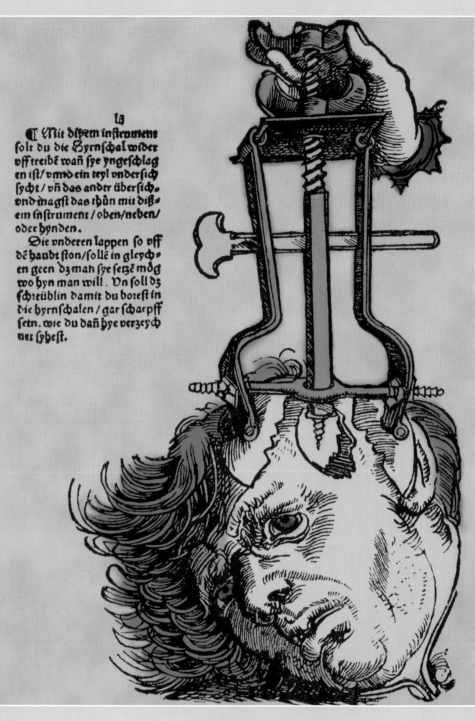

¶ Mit diſem inſtrument
ſolt du die Hyrnſchal wider
off treibē wañ ſye yngeſchlag
en iſt/ vnd ein teyl vnderſich
ſycht/ vñ das andtr überſich.
ond magſt das thůn mit diß
em ſnſtrument / oben/ neben/
oder hynden.

Die vnderen lappen ſo off
dē haudt ſton/ſollē in gleych=
en geen dz man ſye ſetzē mōg
wo hyn man will. Vn ſoll dz
ſchrēüblin damit du boreſt in
die hyrnſchalen / gar ſcharpff
ſetn. wie du dañ hye verzeych
net ſyheſt.

COLOR PLATE #2
The Trepanation of the Skull. After a woodcut by Gerrssdorf's field book of surgery. Undated.
Credit Line: Bettmann/CORBIS

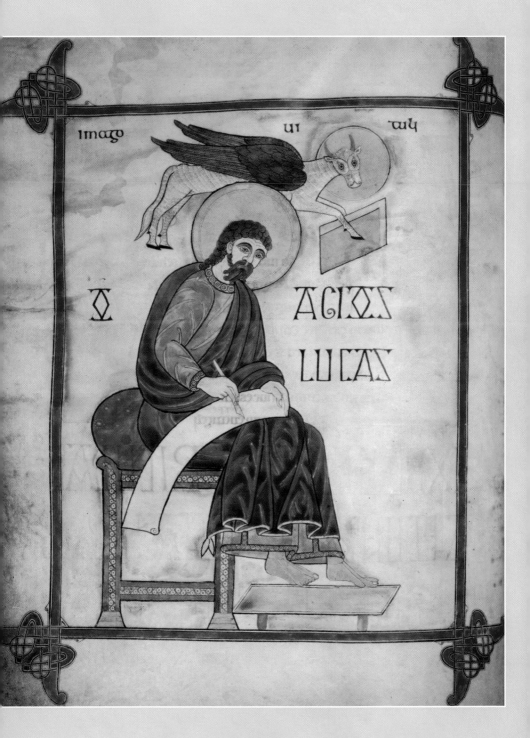

COLOR PLATE #3
Cott Nero DIV f.137v St. Luke's portrait page
Credit Line: The Bridgman Art Library/Getty Images

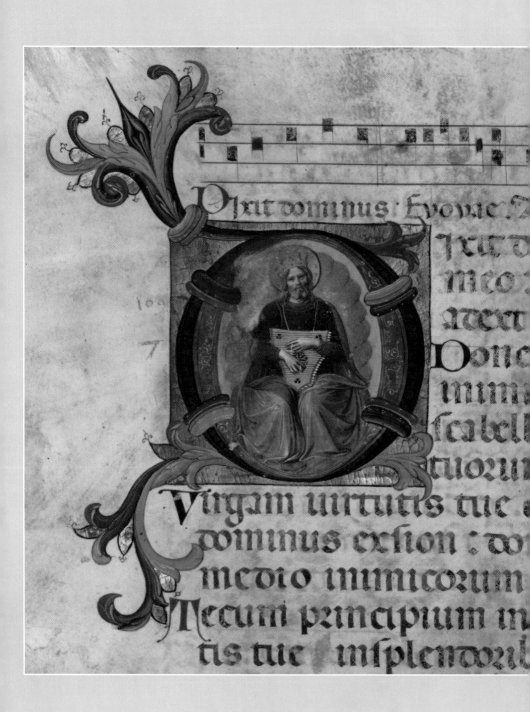

COLOR PLATE #4

Ms 531 f. 169v Historiated initial 'D' depicting King David with his lyre, from a psalter from San Marco with Cenacoli (vellum).
Photographer: Fra Angelico.
Credit Line: The Bridgman Art Library/Getty images

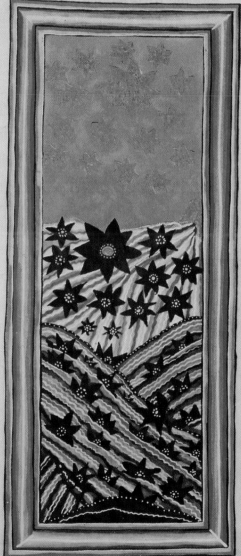

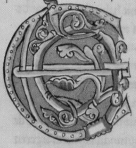

Ego
homo
sumpta
abalus
homim
uis que
ñ sudig
na nomi
nari homo ppr tnsgressione legis
di. cu deberem ee uista & sum inuista.
u qd di creatura sum ipsi gra. que
me etia saluabit. uidi ad orientem.
& ecce illuc conspexi uelut lapidem
unu totu integru unise latitudi
nis atq; altitudinis. habente ferreu
colore. & sup ipsum candida nube.
ac sup ea positu regalem tronum ro
tundu. mquo sedebat quida uiuen
lucidus mirabilis gle. tantq, clarita
tis ut nullaten eu pspicue possem
ituen. habens qsi in pectore suo li
mu nigru & lutulentu. tantq lati
tudinis ut alicu magni hominis
pectus e. circudatu lapidib, pciosis
atq; margaritis. Et de ipso lucido
sedente xrono prendebat magnus
circulus aurei coloris ut aurora. cui
amplitudine nullom cophendere
potui. guans ab oriente ad septento
ne & ad occidente atq; ad meridiem.

COLOR PLATE #5
"Scivias" (Know the ways of the Lord) by the German nun and mystic Hildegard von Bingen (1098–1179). The book, *Codex Rupertsberg*, disappeared during WWII. Transparencies are from a facsimile. Lucifer and his followers shine like bright stars at first, but are extinguished and turn dark as they turn away from God. Romanesque, 12th century. Credit Line: Erich Lessing/Art Resource, NY

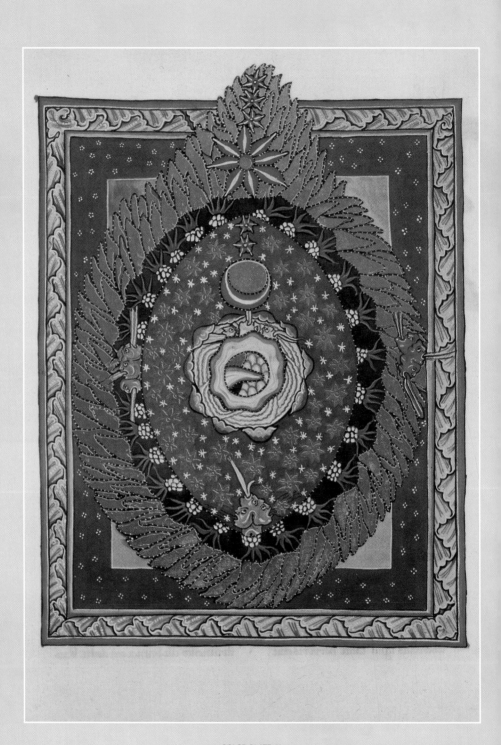

COLOR PLATE #6

"Scivias" (Know the ways of the Lord) by the German nun and mystic Hildegard von Bingen (1098–1179). The book, *Codex Rupertsberg*, disappeared during WWII. Transparencies are from a facsimile. The universe, in the form of an egg; earth with four elements in its center.

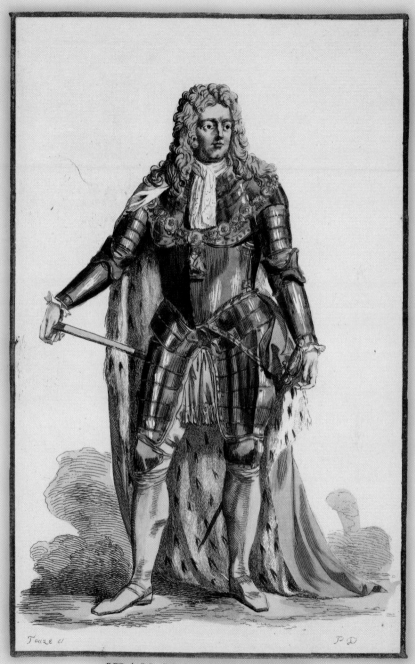

JEAN MARBOUROUGH.

General Anglois.

d'Apres Hondorf.

A Paris chez Duflos le Jeune

A.P.D.R.

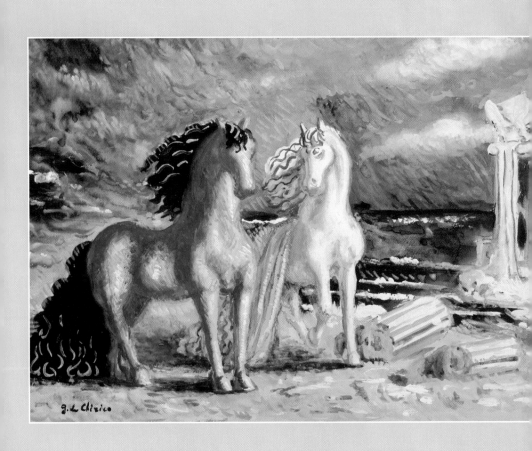

COLOR PLATE #8
Giorgio de Chirico (1888–1978) ARS, NY, Horses. Location: Pinacoteca Provinciale, Bari, Italy
Credit Line: Alinari / Art Resource, NY

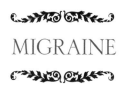

MIGRAINE

everal definitions of migraine have been formulated. We prefer the definition developed by the World Federation of Neurology,[39] "a familial disorder characterized by recurrent attacks of headache widely variable in intensity, frequency, and duration. Attacks are commonly unilateral and are usually associated with anorexia, nausea, and vomiting. In some cases, they are preceded by, or associated with, neurological and mood disturbances."

The types of migraine include migraine with aura, migraine without aura, complicated migraine, and menstrual migraine. The definitive characteristic of migraine with aura is the occurrence of a neurological symptom complex 5 to 30 minutes before the onset of an acute migraine attack. Complicated migraine is described as migraine attacks associated with focal neurological symptoms that may persist after headache disappears. Ophthalmoplegic, hemiplegic, and basilar artery migraine are considered forms of complicated migraine.

Seventy percent of adult migraineurs are female, and 70 percent of those female migraine sufferers will report a menstrual relationship to their acute migraine attacks. Menstrual migraine attacks can occur immediately before, during, or after menses, or at ovulation. Many female migraineurs will report a decrease or complete remission in their headaches after the first trimester of pregnancy.

MIGRAINE

MIGRAINE PATHOGENESIS

"WE CAN DESCRIBE THE THOUGHTS OF HAMLET,
BUT WE CANNOT DESCRIBE A MIGRAINE."

— *Virginia Woolf*

Virginia Woolf (1882 to 1941) made major contributions to modern fiction in her role as a sensitive critic and an important innovator in modern British literature. Through these works, the struggle with her mental disorders and chronic headaches have been known.

Several theories have evolved on the pathogenesis of migraine. In his pioneering work during the 1930s, Harold G.

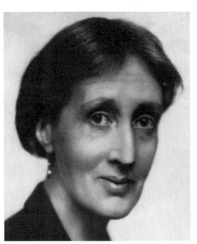

FIGURE 17: Virginia Woolf, ca. 1936
English novelist, critic and essayist Virginia Woolf. She is regarded as one of the great modern innovators of the English novel.
Credit Line: Hulton-Deutsch Collection/Corbis

Wolff identified four dynamic events occurring in a migraine attacks: 1) the warning stage (aura); 2) extracranial vasodilation, which may be the cause of migraine pain; 3) sterile inflammation, which increases pain and prolongs the acute migraine attack; and, 4) secondary muscle contraction. Wolff described migraine as a self-limited neurogenic, sterile inflammation.[40] He believed that

the vasoconstriction occurring during the aura has usually concluded before the extracranial vasodilation begins.

During the 1980s, Lauritzen and Olesen published findings that questioned the theories of Wolff.[41] After injecting
xenon-133, a radioactive isotope, into the carotid artery, they
induced migraine after arteriography. They described a "spreading oligemia," usually beginning in the occipital region and radi-
ating anteriorly. The oligemia continued after the focal symptoms
abated. These investigators concluded the painless aura phase was
possibly secondary to the spreading depression originally
described by the Brazilian neurophysiologist, Leao, and was not
due to the oligemia. In an earlier study, Olesen had noted that the
oligemia did not occur in migraine without aura.[42] The results of
these investigations have been disputed. Skyhøj Olsen's group
have proposed that the "spreading oligemia" observed in cerebral
fluid (CBF) studies during acute migraine with aura may represent an artifact which reflects a gradual decreases of CBF in an
area of constant size.[43] Their findings support the theory that
migraine with aura and migraine without aura are due to the same
disease process, although these two entities vary in the degree of
vasospasm and CBF reduction. A German research group has utilized PET scanning in their investigations. They suggested that
the brain stem is the neurological source of migraine.[44]

MIGRAINE

The clinical features of migraine include unilateral location, recurrent frequency of 2 to 8 times per month, duration of 4 to 24 hours, and varied degree of severity from moderate to incapacitating. Migraine headaches are frequently described as throbbing or pulsating, and associated with nausea, vomiting, and photo- and phonophobia. These headaches are often exacerbated by physical activity.

"DO YOU KNOW WHAT HEMICRANIA IS?
IT IS A HALF HEADACHE AND I HAVE BEEN HAVING ONE
FOR FOUR DAYS NOW. ONE HALF OF MY HEAD, FROM THE TOP
OF MY SKULL TO THE CLEFT OF MY JAW, HAMMERS, BANGS, SIZZLES,
AND SWEARS WHILE THE OTHER HALF, SERENE AND
CONTENT, LOOKS ON AT THE AGONY NEXT DOOR."

— *Rudyard Kipling, letter to a relative, 1896*

Rudyard Kipling (1865 to 1936) was the first English writer to win the Nobel Prize for literature (1907). He was born in Bombay, India, and educated in England. His poems and short stories are celebrations of British imperialism. From 1882 to 1889, he returned to his birthplace to write for Indian newspapers. Returning to England, he gained success with the publication of his semi-autobiographical novel, *The Light That Failed*.

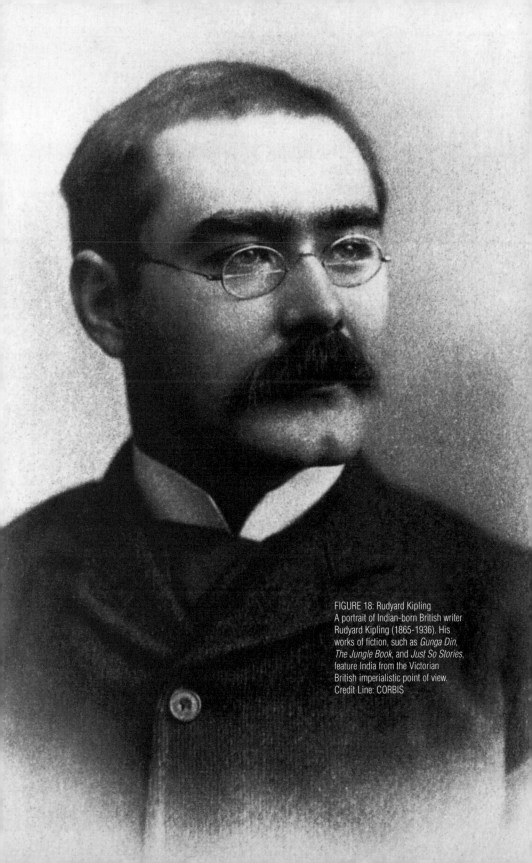

FIGURE 18: Rudyard Kipling
A portrait of Indian-born British writer
Rudyard Kipling (1865-1936). His
works of fiction, such as *Gunga Din*,
The Jungle Book, and *Just So Stories*,
feature India from the Victorian
British imperialistic point of view.
Credit Line: CORBIS

Many of his works relate to his Indian experiences: *The Jungle Books* (1894 and 1895), *Kim* (1901), and the *Just So Stories* (1902). A visit to the United States prompted the classic, *Captains Courageous*. Kipling used a variety of settings, such as India, London, the sea, and the jungle, to promote his ideas of duty, the importance of law, and the righteousness of British colonialism.

His description of a migraine attack is right "on the mark." Migraine derives its name from the French word for hemicrania, meaning "half-a-head." Typically, a migraine only affects one side of the head, although it can switch sides during an attack. The duration of migraine characteristically ranges from 4 to 24 hours, although some attacks will continue for over one day and may be termed "status migraine." Kipling's descriptions of the pain are very illustrative of the throbbing quality of a migraine attack. Often, the site of the pain is warm to the touch. Kipling also provides us with a depiction of the absence of symptoms on the side opposite from the headache.

One noted migraine sufferer was Thomas Jefferson (1743 to 1826), the 3rd President of the United States, an astute scholar of the sciences, poetry, and politics, and a prolific writer. Jefferson was the primary author of the *Declaration of Independence* — and on his tombstone, he scripted his own dedication, *"author of the Declaration of American Independence, of the Statute of Virginia for religious freedom, and Father of the University of Virginia."* Jefferson had requested *"not another word more."*

Similar to many of his peers, Jefferson kept a daily journal, affording historians tremendous insight into his activities, beliefs, and personal life. Without the benefit of telephone and

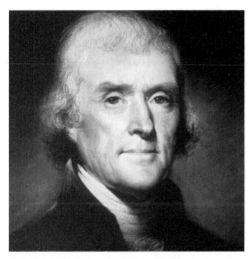

FIGURE 19: Portrait of President Thomas Jefferson by Rembrandt Peale. An 1800 portrait of Thomas Jefferson (1743–1826), the third president of the United States. He served as President from 1801–1809.
Credit Line: Bettmann/CORBIS

e-mail, Jefferson was a profuse correspondent with family, friends, politicians, and his legion of admirers. In a letter from 1786,[45] Jefferson revealed that *"The Art of life is the avoiding of pain."* Through his journals, we know that his migraine attacks occurred at intervals of several years. He described, in correspondence from 1790, *"an attack of the periodical headache, which came on me about a week ago rendering me unable as yet to write or read without great pain."*

During the last year of his presidency (1808), Jefferson reflected on his problem in a letter to his granddaughter, Cornelia Randolph:

"I MENTIONED IN MY LETTER OF LAST WEEK TO ELLEN, THAT I WAS UNDER AN ATTACK OF PERIODICAL HEADACHE. THIS IS THE TENTH DAY. IT HAS BEEN VERY MODERATE, AND YESTERDAY DID NOT LAST MORE THAN THREE HOURS."

Jefferson refused to focus on his headaches and continued with his extraordinary life.

Migraine typically starts in adolescence and during the early twenties. It rarely starts over the age of 40 years. Characteristically, migraine gradually diminishes and disappears as a person ages. Jefferson was no exception. When he was 76, in 1819, Jefferson replied to a correspondent who had inquired about the state of his health, that: *"A periodical headache has afflicted me occasionally, once, perhaps, in six or eight years, for two or three weeks at a time, which seems now to have left me."* Typical of migraine, the headaches that bothered Jefferson throughout his life, seemed to abate as he aged.

The following quote serves to illustrate that well-known characteristic of migraine:

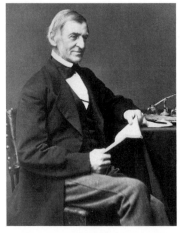

FIGURE 20: Ralph Waldo Emerson (1803–1882), the American poet and essayist, author of *English Traits* (1856) and *Society and Solitude* (1872). Credit Line: Hulton-Deutsch Collection/CORBIS

AT FIFTY YEARS, 'TIS SAID, AFFLICTED CITIZENS LOSE THEIR SICK HEADACHES. SOCIETY AND SOLITUDE, "OLD AGE"

— *Ralph Waldo Emerson*

Emerson (1803 to 1882) was an American essayist, lecturer, and poet. With the above quote, it appears he was an astute observer of headache — and most probably was a migraine sufferer himself.

For women with migraine, in whom 70 percent report a menstrual relationship to their acute attacks, the headaches usually disappear after menopause. Some elderly patients with aura symptoms preceding the headache may report experiencing the aura without the succeeding headache. Emerson also notes the "sick headaches" — a common name for migraine. This alias can be attributed to the associated symptoms of nausea and vomiting that usually accompany an acute migraine attack. Migraine is often depicted as a "sick" headache. Associated symptoms of migraine include nausea, vomiting, photo- and phonophobia, dizziness, tinnitus, and blurred vision. The occurrence of these associated symptoms may influence the selection of abortive and pain-relieving agents, as well as the route of administration.

In childhood migraine, the sex distribution is equal but a female predominance (60 to 70 percent) is noted after puberty. The life and work of Charles Darwin (1809 to 1882) had a profound effect on both science and theology of the 19th century. His theory of evolution revolutionized biology with the publication of *On the Origin of Species* (1859) and *The Descent of Man* (1871). His headaches reportedly started during his twenties — he experienced a severe headache a few days prior to his marriage to a cousin, Emma Wedgewood. According to records, Darwin did not fear marriage but rather the formality of the ceremony, *"As the excruciating moment drew close, Charles' usual symptoms appeared."* Darwin wrote to his fiancee:

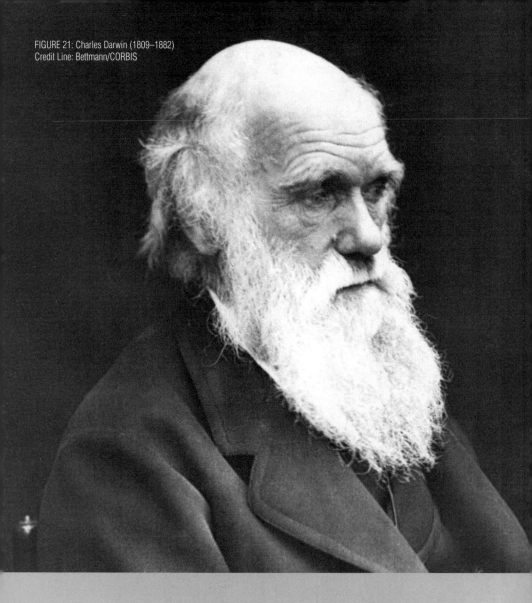

"My last two days in London, when I wanted to
have most leisure, were rendered very uncomfortable
by a bad headache, which continued two days and two
nights, so that I doubted whether it ever meant to go
and allow me to be married."[46]

This occurrence of a headache attack prior to a special event is typical of migraine, which seems to have a will of its own. Frequently, migraine sufferers will manage to get through an event, perhaps a daughter's wedding, with the fear of an impending headache constantly present. At the end of this joyous, yet stressful occasion, a severe headache will manifest. Darwin himself could not attend the funeral of his father — Charles was in the throes of a severe migraine attack.

Darwin's headaches continued, usually triggered by the slightest deviation from his normal routine. His wife and children learned to live with them, adapting to life with a headache sufferer, *"a pall settled over his family. The children played in a depressed hush."*

Darwin described his headache condition as his *"hereditary weakness."* Three of his children inherited his headaches. Up to 70 percent of migraineurs will report a family history of similar headaches. A family history of depression may be elicited in those patients with chronic tension-type headaches.

Some researchers believe that Darwin was suffering from depression. In one letter, Darwin writes that *"We have just returned home after spending five weeks in Ulswater; the scenery is quite charming, but I cannot walk, and everything tires me, even seeing scenery . . . What I shall do with my few remaining years I can hardly tell, I have everything to make me happy and contented, but life has become very wearisome to me."* Pickering in *Creative Malady* challenges this theory of depression, noting that unlike the typical depressed patient, Darwin was not prevented from performing tasks during the supposed long periods of depression.[46] During his years as a recluse, Darwin was productive in his writings.

His marriage to Emma certainly helped him be productive as he withdrew from society. Before their wedding, Darwin experienced occasional illnesses. Following the nuptials, he became an invalid — unable to attend scientific meetings and social events at friends' homes, as well as avoiding visitors at his own home. Emma served as his shield, allowing him the time and tranquility to produce. If social interactions made Charles ill, then a move to the country was in order. Emma also enjoyed caring for invalids. This phenomena has been described as the "concubine syndrome." It is most often seen in female patients — their illness is used for secondary gain by a significant other (spouse, parent, lover, child). The illness makes the victim totally

EVEN IN THE LAST FEW WEEKS OF HIS LIFE, DARWIN CONTINUED TO SUFFER FROM THE HEADACHES.

dependent on their caregiver. This scenario is not limited to headache and can be seen in many chronic states. Emma Darwin was a facilitator of Charles' illness, whether it be imaginary or real.

In his later years, his illnesses improved — refuting the claim that his ailments were due to infection or other organic syndrome. Darwin was able to become even more productive in the last decade of his life. At age 73 years, in 1882, he died of coronary heart disease. Darwin had suffered a heart attack and lingered for several weeks. Even in the last few weeks of his life, Darwin continued to suffer from the headaches. His son, Frank, wrote in a letter to Thomas Huxley, that on the eve of Darwin's death, *"He remained in a condition of terrible faintness and suffered very much from overpowering nausea, interrupted by retchings. He more than once said, if I could but die."*

THE MIGRAINE PRODROME

Migraine with aura is defined by the occurrence of prodromal neurological symptoms. The most frequent aura symptoms are visual in nature, such as blurred vision, distorted vision, defects in the visual field, and seeing bright lights or jagged lines. Other prodromal symptoms include ocular paralysis or hemiparesis. The aura symptoms will usually continue for 5 to 30 minutes prior to the onset of the headache. Older patients may experience the prodromal symptoms without the occurrence of a headache.

Some patients with migraine will report vague, premonitory symptoms prior to a headache, starting as early as 48 hours before a migraine attack. These symptoms include hunger, fatigue, a burst of energy, and anorexia.

❦

"I'M VERY BRAVE GENERALLY," HE WENT ON IN A LOW VOICE: "ONLY TODAY I HAPPEN TO HAVE A HEADACHE."

❦

— *Tweedle Dum, Through the Looking Glass, Lewis Carroll* (1872)

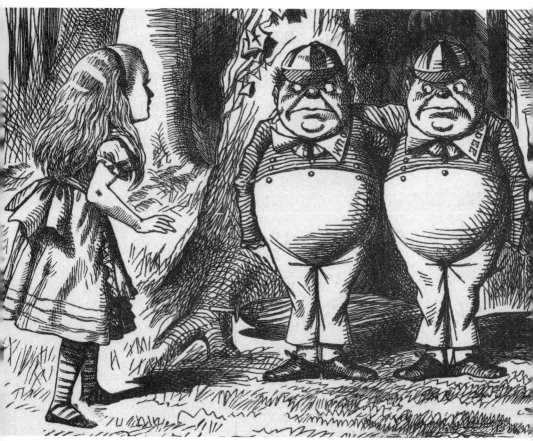

FIGURE 22: Tweedledum and Tweedledee, by John Tenniel. Illustration of Alice and the twins Tweedledee and Tweedledum from *Through the Looking Glass*, the sequel to *Alice's Adventures in Wonderland*, both written by Lewis Carroll. Credit Line: Bettmann/CORBIS

This quote from the beloved children's classic was penned by the English clergyman, mathematician, and author, Charles Lutwidge Dodgson (1832 to 1898), under the pseudonym, Lewis Carroll. Dodgson was the son of a clergyman and was the oldest of 11 children. He attended Rugby School and graduated from Christ Church College in Oxford in 1854. His first novel, *Alice in Wonderland*, was produced as a gift for Alice Liddell, one of the daughters of the dean of his college. His pen name was created by translating his first two names into Latin, *Carolus Lodovicus*, and then anglicizing them into Lewis Carroll.

Carroll remained at Christ Church College after graduation, lecturing on mathematics and authoring treatises and guides for students. He was ordained as a deacon in 1861, but was never ordained as a priest. Carroll had a stammer, rendering preaching difficult. As a mathematician, he was an expert in Euclidian geometry. Carroll used logic as a game rather than an instrument for testing reason. When *Alice in Wonderland* is analyzed from a mathematical viewpoint, it corresponds to a real and complex chess game. The movements and adventures of the characters (Alice, the Red Queen, the White Knight) represent actual moves on a chessboard. One of his hobbies was photography, and he became especially expert at photographing children, including Alice Lidell and her sisters.

Carroll was acquainted with many gentlemen from upper-class society, including physicians. His interest in medicine and in children led to his bequeathing a perpetual endowment of a bed in the Children's Hospital in London. From his diaries, we know

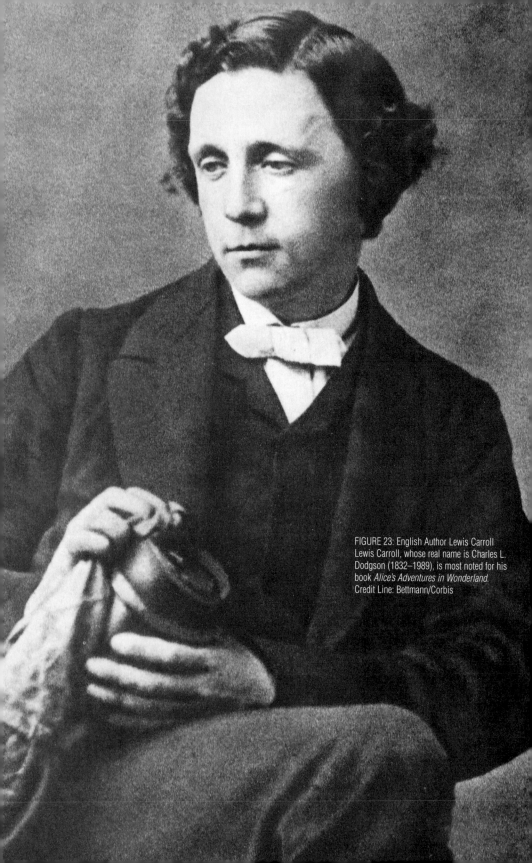

FIGURE 23: English Author Lewis Carroll
Lewis Carroll, whose real name is Charles L.
Dodgson (1832–1989), is most noted for his
book *Alice's Adventures in Wonderland*.
Credit Line: Bettmann/Corbis

that for many years, Carroll suffered from what he described as "bilious headaches." He experienced aura symptoms of eye disturbances and fortification spectra. It should be noted that his descriptions of his headaches appeared in his diaries many years after publication of his children's novels. He never provides any detailing of body image hallucinations although it is believed that the body distortions in his works were features of his own migraine attacks and auras.

The "Alice-in-Wonderland" syndrome, which refers to a distortion of body image as a migraine aura, was first described by Lippman in 1952,[47] although the name was not given to this phenomena until 1955 by Todd.[48] Lippman reported on seven patients with migraine who related aura symptoms of altered perceptions of their body image. In some patients, the headache never appeared and the hallucination was the entire attack. One of Lippman's patients described a sensation of her left ear as "ballooning out 6 inches or more." Another patient noted "I felt that I was very tall. When walking down the street, I would think I would be able to look down on the tops of others'

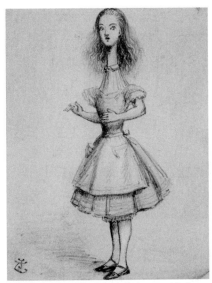

FIGURE 24: Alice in Wonderland: *Curiouser and Curiouser* by John Tenniel
Credit Line: Christie's Images/CORBIS

heads, and it was very frightening and annoying not to see as I was feeling. The sensation was so real that when I would see myself in a window or full-length mirror, it was quite a shock to realize that I was still my normal height of under 5 feet."

How does this relate to Alice in Wonderland? In one famous scene, Alice finds a bottle marked "Drink Me," and the liquid caused her to shrink. After she eats a piece of cake marked "Eat Me," she begins to grow. Her size continues to fluctuate throughout her encounters with the Mad Hatter, the Cheshire Cat, the Walrus, the Carpenter, and other characters. Another of Lippman's patients recalled feeling short and wide as she walked along, similar to the charac-

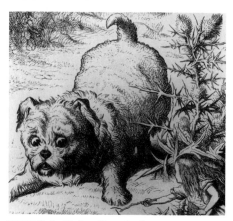

FIGURE 25: One Big Dog. Alice and a giant puppy.
From *Alice in Wonderland* by Lewis Carroll.
Alice Through The Looking Glass, 1st Edition, pub. 1872
Illustration by John Tenniel
Credit Line: Rischgitz/Getty Images

ters from Carroll — Tweedle Dee or Tweedle Dum.

Arnold Friedman was a prominent headache researcher and founder of the headache clinic at Montefiore Hospital in the Bronx. His reports on posttraumatic headache in returning GIs from World War II changed many of the current ideas on this syndrome. Doctor Friedman also developed a keen interest in the history of migraine, and particularly the citations of this malady in literature. According to Friedman, the character of the White Rabbit provides us an example of the migraine personality.[22] When we first encounter this character, on the very first page of *Alice in Wonderland*, he hurries by anxiously, muttering, "Oh dear! Oh dear! I shall be too late!" The rabbit continues this behavior throughout the story, fretting needlessly, dropping things when he is spoken to, and apparently living in dire fear of the terrifying Duchess and the imperious Queen of Hearts.

ALL AT ONCE, ON MY RIGHT, ON THE OTHER SIDE OF THE STREET, I SAW ON THE FIRST FLOOR BALCONY OF A HOUSE A GREAT BLACK PALL FLYING IN THE WIND. IT WAS LIKE A FLASH OF DARKNESS IN THE BRIGHT LIGHT THAT FLOODED EVERYTHING. I FELT A SUDDEN ANGUISH AND TERRIBLE PRESENTIMENT.

— Memoirs, Georgio de Chirico, 1971

De Chirico (1888 to 1978) was born in Greece, the son of a Sicilian railroad engineer. He studied in Athens and Munich, and moved to his father's native Italy in 1909. De Chirico is considered an important forerunner of surrealism in 20th century painting. The philosophies of Nietzsche and Schopenhauer — noted migraine sufferers — influenced his early painting. His work combined remnants of classical antiquity with modern ideas from northern Europe. His first exhibitions from 1911 to 1915, in Paris, included enigmatic, dreamlike paintings. During this interval in Paris, he became acquainted with Picasso and the cubists.

His friend, Guillaume Appollinaire, the symbolist poet, garnered the description of de Chirico's independent style as "metaphysical art" (see color plate #8).

In his memoirs, de Chirico noted experiencing several complaints.[49] He described a triad of symptoms — motion sickness, abdominal pain, and vomiting — suggesting a periodic syndrome. His presentation reflects the syndrome of abdominal migraine, a form of acephalic migraine. Some patients will complain of these gastrointestinal symptoms in the absence of a headache, and the symptoms will occur periodically similar to migraine attacks. In de Chirico, his symptoms were effectively treated with sedatives. On two occasions during his early adulthood, he complained of headaches that were terrible and extremely painful.

But in the context of this book, our interest in de Chirico are the visual symptoms which had influenced his art. The above description of his aura reflected an incident that occurred on the day of his father's death. In his semi-autobiographical novel, *Hebdomeros*, de Chirico, published in 1964, noted:[50]

He sensed also that he was going to witness inexplicable phenomena . . . Until then everything had gone well, but now the cock, or rather this silhouette, this shadow of a cock was becoming gradually obsessive and began to occupy a preponderant place in the countryside and to play a part in the life of this modest and tranquil spot. Now the silhouette moved downwards; at the same time it moved upwards; acting as a corrosive, it consumed the steeple on one side while on the other it broke into the sky by standing out against it and unfolding there with a slow and inexplicable regularity.

This passage described negative scotomata — that is a defect is occurring in the center of the visual field, gradually spreading towards the periphery. De Chirico provides us with a characteristic portrayal of symptoms of aura. The gradual "march of symptoms" distinguishes migraine aura from that related to other causes. De Chirico also experienced positive scotomata — visual symptoms which include sparking, dazzling, flickering, or dancing lights:

BUT HOW CONFUSED IT ALL WAS, GOOD HEAVENS! DELIGHTFUL RIBBONS, FLAMES WITHOUT WARMTH, THRUST FORWARD LIKE THIRSTY TONGUES, DISTURBING BUBBLES, LINES DRAWN WITH 'MAESTRIA' WHICH HE THOUGHT HAD LONG BEEN FORGOTTEN, DELICATE WAVES, OBSTINATE AND ISOCHRONUS, MOVED CONTINUOUSLY UP AND UP TOWARDS HIS BEDROOM CEILING. IT ALL WENT AWAY IN A CORKSCREW FORMATION, OR ELSE IN REGULAR ZIGZAGS, OR ELSE IN STRICTLY PERPENDICULAR FASHION RESEMBLING PIKES CARRIED BY A DISCIPLINED TROOP ... HEBDOMEROS, FORTIFIED BY MANY EXPERIENCES, IMAGINED THAT THE SPIRITUAL FEVER WHICH HAD LAID HIM LOW AT THIS MOMENT WOULD LAST NO LONGER THAN ANY OF THE PRECEDING ONES. SINCE HE SUPPOSED ALL THIS WOULD HAPPEN TO HIM AGAIN, HE LINGERED LATE THAT EVENING AND HIS THOUGHT WENT BEYOND THE PERMITTED LIMITS.

In addition to the literary descriptions of his pain, De Chirico contributed many paintings which suggest the symptoms of migraine aura. He illustrated Cocteau's "Mythologie," with the jagged effect of the water similar to the advancing edge of a scotoma. A painting from 1969, "The Return to the Castle," depicts a knight nearing a fortress with a spiky edge, similar to the fortification spectra. A lithograph completed in 1930, "Calligrammes," shows a black sun motif intruding into an interior scene. De Chirico painted throughout his 90-year life but his best work is considered that produced in the early part of this century. He was productive despite his pain, and his work affords those interested in headache to have both literary and visual depictions of the pain and visual phenomena of migraine.

DO NOT UNDERVALUE THE HEADACHE. WHILE IT IS AT ITS
SHARPEST IT SEEMS A BAD INVESTMENT; BUT WHEN RELIEF BEGINS,
THE UNEXPIRED REMAINDER IS WORTH $4 A MINUTE.

— *Following the Equator, Volume II, Chapter 18, Pudd'nhead
Wilson's New Calendar. Mark Twain (Samuel L. Clemens).*

Mark Twain is the pseudonym of Samuel Clemens (1835 to 1910). Twain was the first fiction writer to truly reflect the American talent. His description of headache is exceptionally accurate. If he was a headache sufferer during his many years of wandering, Twain would understand the futility of some relief agents. The amount subscribed for the period of relief, "$4 a minute," was a hefty sum during Twain's lifetime. His description of the denouement of a headache reflects on the post-headache surges of energy that could be considered a "postdrome" of the acute attack. The majority of migraine attacks are terminated by sleep, which could be a brief period or a deep sleep lasting several hours. A postdromal period has been described by many migraine patients. The symptoms may be vague with the patient indicating that "I just feel differ-ent." Weakness and listlessness may be present, particularly if the attack is accompanied by vomiting and diarrhea. Depression may be observed with the headache sufferer not able to perform any activity due to impaired concentration, difficulty reading, fatigue, and irritability. These patients may limit their physical activities and avoid exertion.

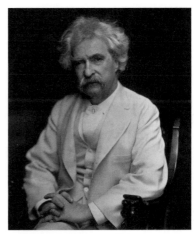

FIGURE 26: Mark Twain
Credit Line: CORBIS

Many patients will report feeling absolutely normal after the pain is resolved, and may actually note a sense of enthusiasm, feeling ebullient and energetic.

MIGRAINE PERSONALITY

The subject of a migraine personality has been a topic of debate for decades. Migraineurs are often described as compulsive, perfectionistic, and as building environments too great to handle.

Arthur Schopenhauer (1788 to 1860), the German philosopher, has been identified as a migraine sufferer, although evidence is lacking. However, some of his commentaries hint at a migraine pattern. If he did not experience migraine, Schopenhauer was cognizant of migraine's characteristics. In *Counsels and Maxims*, he wrote:

❧

" . . . IN PROPORTION AS . . . CONSCIOUSNESS ASCENDS,
PAIN ALSO INCREASES, AND REACHES ITS HIGHEST DEGREE
IN MAN. AND THEN, AGAIN, THE MORE DISTINCTLY A MAN KNOWS —
THE MORE INTELLIGENT HE IS — THE MORE PAIN HE HAS; THE MAN
WHO IS GIFTED WITH GENIUS SUFFERS MOST OF ALL."

❧

Schopenhauer believed that you could escape from pain by subordinating the will to a greater endeavor.

His remarks on the intelligence of the man in pain has also been described by Harold G. Wolff who noted that the childhood of migraine sufferers revealed that more than half were delicate, shy, withdrawn, and extremely obedient.[40] These children often had an unusual stubbornness or inflexibility. This characteristic was in contrast with the courteous, gracious, polite behavior shown in public. The same person could be obstinate, defiant, or even rebellious. Frequently, out of frustration, these children would throw temper tantrums. Their parents and teachers also found them sensitive, trustworthy, and energetic, and were often given responsibilities at an early age. During their adolescence,

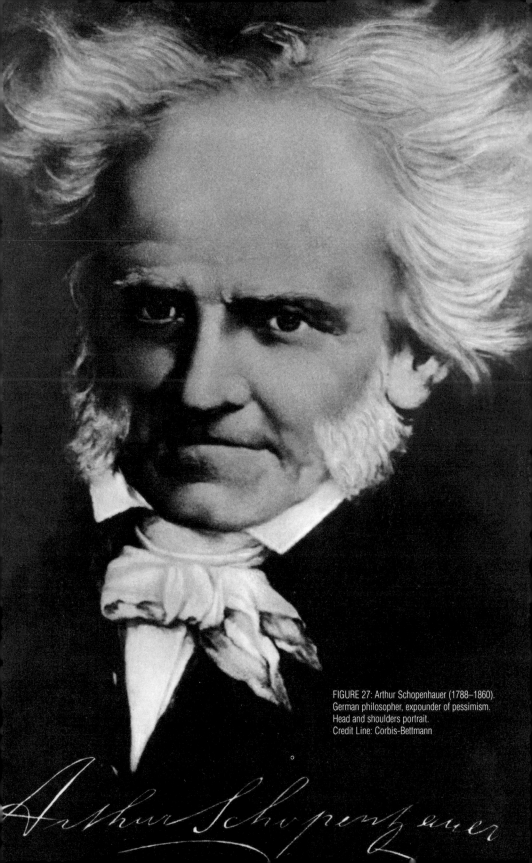

FIGURE 27: Arthur Schopenhauer (1788–1860).
German philosopher, expounder of pessimism.
Head and shoulders portrait.
Credit Line: Corbis-Bettmann

these young migraine sufferers were frequently preoccupied with moralistic and ethical problems, particularly with sex.

In adulthood, 90% of these headache sufferers were ambitious and preoccupied with achievements and success. The adult migraineurs were conscientious, persistent, and exacting, but could be unforgiving and inflexible. Their goal was to bring order to any situation. Teachers, coworkers, and family members described them as meticulous and hard-working.

MIGRAINE IS LEAST COMMON IN HEALTHY MALES,
RESTRICTED TO THE SEXUAL TIME OF LIFE, OCCURS AFTER
AN ACCUMULATION OF INTERNAL OR EXTERNAL STIMULI,
IS CHARACTERIZED BY PERIODICITY OF OUTBREAKS AND
RESULTS FROM COMPLEX AETIOLOGY . . .

— Sigmund Freud, 1885

Sigmund Freud (1856 to 1939), father of psychoanalysis, philosopher, physician, and migraine sufferer. He was born in Freiberg, Moravia — now part of the Czech Republic — to a Jewish woolen merchant and his second wife. When he was 4 years of age, the family moved to Leipzig, Germany, and then to Vienna, Austria. As so many of the headache sufferers described in this text, Freud was a precocious child, reading Shakespeare by the age of 8 years. His insight into emotions and human motivation were first demonstrated in letters he composed during his adolescence. At first he considered a career in law, but then prompted by an essay on nature by Goethe, Freud determined to pursue medical research. He started medical school at age 17, but did not finish until age 25, in 1881, due to his interest in zoology and marine biology, and extra years spent working at Brücke's Physiological Institute on the histology (study of tissues) of the nervous system. In 1886, after marrying Martha Bernays, he realized that medical research would not be conducive to supporting a family. Freud then turned to the clinical practice of neurology.

Freud had the opportunity to study with the famous neurologist, Jean Martin Charcot, in Paris and was exposed to the use of therapeutic hypnosis. Freud translated Charcot's work into German. This experience with Charcot, coupled with the successful use of this therapy by Josef Breuer in hysteria, sparked Freud's interest in this condition. He used Breuer's "cathartic method" in his practice and, with Breuer, published *Studies in Hysteria* which described their "talking cure." This is considered to be the beginning of psychoanalysis. Freud's belief that sexuality was the central focus of neurosis was of no interest to Breuer. Freud eventually discarded hypnosis and with his patients' cooperation, he used "free association" discussions which enabled the physician to observe the unconsciously motivated resistance of a patient to

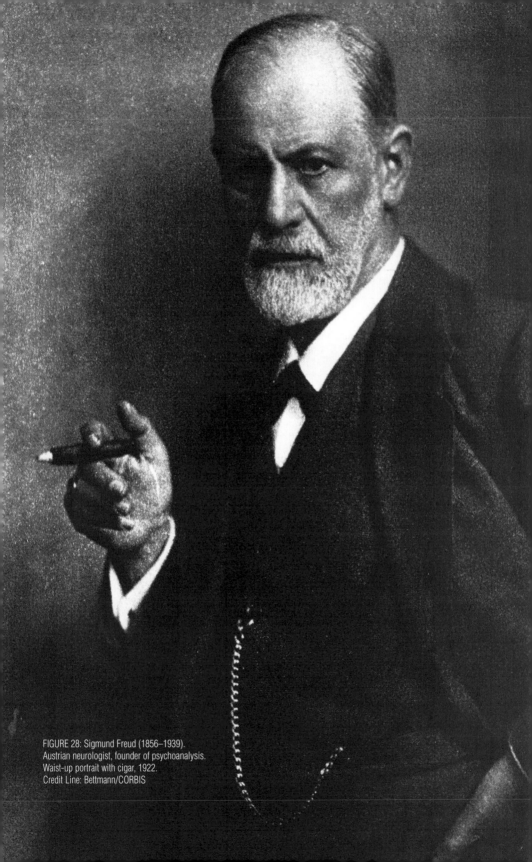

FIGURE 28: Sigmund Freud (1856–1939).
Austrian neurologist, founder of psychoanalysis.
Waist-up portrait with cigar, 1922.
Credit Line: Bettmann/CORBIS

express repressed thoughts and memories, particularly sexual ideas. Via this approach, Freud discovered transference "— the unconscious shift of feelings associated with individual's in the patient's past — to the therapist."

With the dissolution of his collaboration with Breuer, and the death of his father in 1896, Freud began a period of self-analysis. He began to explore, with the help of Wilhelm Fliess, his dreams and fantasies for clues to his childhood sexual passions. In a letter to Fliess in 1899, he referred to his headaches:

"... MY DEPRESSION LEFT ME, NOT AFTER ONE MIGRAINE,
BUT AFTER A WHOLE SERIES OF SUCH STATES."

The following year, he noted that:

"... MY HEALTH HAS BEEN EXCELLENT —
REGULATED BY A SLIGHT MIGRAINE ON SUNDAYS."

Arnold Friedman related the precipitant of Freud's attack was probably the Christian Sabbath.[22] Freud battled antisemitism throughout his life. It is believed that his failure to gain a more prestigious appointment, prompting his joining the staff of the Vienna Children's Hospital during the early 1890s, was due to his religion. His exile from Austria in 1937 was due to the escalating violence against the Jews in the Third Reich.

In 1900, Freud published what he considered his greatest book, *The Interpretation of Dreams*. Although initially ignored, this text gradually drew interest, and he developed a group around him who wished to study with the physician and apply his discoveries to clinical practice. Although some of his early followers, such as Alfred Adler and Carl Jung, eventually developed their own schools of psychology, his impact on this discipline is immeasurable.

During the next decades of his life, Freud developed the technique to psychoanalytic treatment of neuroses, and developed guidelines for this therapy. Due to Freud's work, an entire new field of scientific research was established that investigated our emotional world. He was not universally accepted, and some of his findings aroused hostility among his colleagues. Following World War I, Freud was diagnosed with cancer of the jaw, and underwent 33 surgeries, and 17 years of chronic pain and disability. He did gain some measure of recognition, with receipt of the Goethe Prize for Literature in 1930, and election to the Royal Society in 1936. When the Nazis occupied Austria, Freud moved to England where he died on September 23, 1939.

Migraine Triggers

When not preoccupied with psychoanalysis, Freud sought to understand the causes of his migraine attacks. In a letter to his fiancee in May, 1885, Freud wrote:

"I WAS SUFFERING FROM MIGRAINE, THE THIRD ATTACK THIS WEEK INCIDENTALLY, ALTHOUGH I WAS OTHERWISE IN EXCELLENT HEALTH. I SUSPECT THE TARTAR SAUCE I HAD FOR LUNCH [. . .] DISAGREED WITH ME. I TOOK SOME COCAINE, WATCHED THE MIGRAINE VANISH AT ONCE, WENT ON WRITING MY PAPER AS WELL AS A LETTER [. . .] BUT I WAS SO WOUND UP THAT I HAD TO GO ON WORKING AND WRITING AND COULDN'T GET TO SLEEP BEFORE 4 IN THE MORNING. TODAY I AM IN FINE FETTLE AGAIN [. . .]."

In this episode, Freud identifies a trigger to his migraine attack — Tartar sauce. The topic of diet and headache has long been debated. Despite many investigations failing to determine positive allergy testing for headache, including one of the author's own clinical experience, he (Diamond) has observed many patients relating food triggers for their headache attacks. Many migraineurs will note that chocolate or cheese will precipitate a headache. Food items that contain what we call "vasoactive substances" are often linked to headaches. These substances, such as tyramine and phenylethylamine, will cause the blood vessels to dilate in sensitive individuals. The suspect Tartar sauce of Freud's tale, probably contained vinegar — a fermented substance. Other fermented foods (pickles, yogurt, wine), aged cheese, and sausages are often linked to headaches. Nitrates, agents recognized as dilating blood vessels, are added to meats to preserve the red food coloring — for example, hot dogs and cold cuts (bologna, salami).

Patients consuming excessive amounts of caffeine, whether in beverages or analgesics, will experience a withdrawal headache when the caffeine is skipped or omitted. Other patients will consistently complain of a headache when traveling to higher altitudes or during changes in barometric pressure. Migraine patients appear to be particularly susceptible to changes in sleep habits or meal schedules.

COMPLICATED MIGRAINE

One of his biographers called Freud a "martyr to migraine." Through his writings, we do not know if Freud experienced the associated complaints of nausea and vomiting with his headaches. However, we do know that he experienced neurological symptoms with an attack:

❧

"THE MILD ATTACKS OF MIGRAINE FROM WHICH I STILL SUFFER, USUALLY ANNOUNCE THEMSELVES HOURS IN ADVANCE BY MY FORGETTING NAMES, AND AT THE HEIGHT OF THESE ATTACKS, . . . IT FREQUENTLY HAPPENS THAT ALL PROPER NAMES GO OUT OF MY HEAD. . . . SLIPS OF THE TONGUE DO REALLY OCCUR WITH PARTICULAR FREQUENCY WHEN ONE IS TIRED, HAS A HEADACHE OR IS THREATENED WITH MIGRAINE. IN THE SAME CIRCUMSTANCES PROPER NAMES ARE EASILY FORGOTTEN. SOME PEOPLE ARE ACCUSTOMED TO RECOGNIZE THE APPROACH OF AN ATTACK OF MIGRAINE WHEN PROPER NAMES ESCAPE THEM IN THIS WAY."

❧

Migraine attacks that are associated with neurological symptoms — confusion, loss of feelings in the extremities, blindness, difficulties with memory — are termed complicated migraine. Although very few migraine sufferers will ever experience these associated symptoms, their occurrence is very frightening to the individual. Usually, the symptoms will disappear when the headache recedes, but at times, the neurological symptoms will persist. In one form of complicated migraine, basilar artery migraine, the headache sufferer will appear very confused and may be considered under the influence of drugs. Typically, the patient with basilar artery migraine is a young female (adolescents or in their early twenties) and, if brought to an emergency department, may be admitted to a drug rehabilitation unit or to a psychiatric unit. Migraine will be diagnosed if someone can provide a previous history of headaches in the individual or in the patient's family. The name, basilar artery migraine, is related to the site of the headache, at the back of the head and affecting the basilar artery.

Freud's first coherent review of migraine was published in 1895 as a review of a monograph on migraine by PJ Mobius. One of the topics that peaked Freud's interest was migraine equivalents. Freud defined migraine equivalents as attacks with symptoms different from those of migraine. They are distinguished by their mode of occurrence, the course of the attack, and their eventual replacement by migraine headaches. Freud identified three forms of migraine equivalents, according to the areas of the body affected by these symptoms — abdominal migraine, back migraine, and heart migraine. Abdominal migraine, often observed in children, occurs with the same periodic nature of migraine headaches with the patient suffering regular bouts of abdominal pain, nausea, and vomiting. The other forms of migraine equivalents refer to periodic episodes of pain in areas such as the back and chest. Their onset and occurrence are linked to migraine when the pain leaves the original area and in later years, actually evolves as a periodic headache.

AT FIRST EVERY SMALL APPREHENSION IS MAGNIFIED, EVERY ANXIETY A POUNDING TERROR. THEN THE PAIN COMES, AND I CONCENTRATE ONLY ON THAT. RIGHT THERE IS THE USEFULNESS OF THE MIGRAINE, THERE IN THAT IMPOSED YOGA, THE CONCENTRATION ON THE PAIN. FOR WHEN THE PAIN RECEDES, TEN OR TWELVE HOURS LATER, EVERYTHING GOES WITH IT, ALL THE HIDDEN RESENTMENTS, ALL THE VAIN ANXIETIES. THE MIGRAINE HAS ACTED AS A CIRCUIT BREAKER, AND THE FUSES HAVE EMERGED INTACT.

– Joan Didion

Joan Didion (1934–) is an American novelist and essayist — and a definite migraine sufferer. Her first novel, *Play It As It Lays*, published in 1970, portrays a woman whose life reflects the banality of society. Her lack of exposition characterizes her style as seen in *A Book of Common Prayer*, published in 1977. She has written screen plays, nonfiction, and essay collections, such as *After Henry*.

In her quoted narrative of an acute migraine, Didion relates the actual sense of relief at the end of a headache. The events which led up to the onset of the pain are resolved, and the headache sufferer can once again enjoy life. Unfortunately, the migraineur knows that the headache will again return — and the inherent anxiety about headache occurrence will persist.

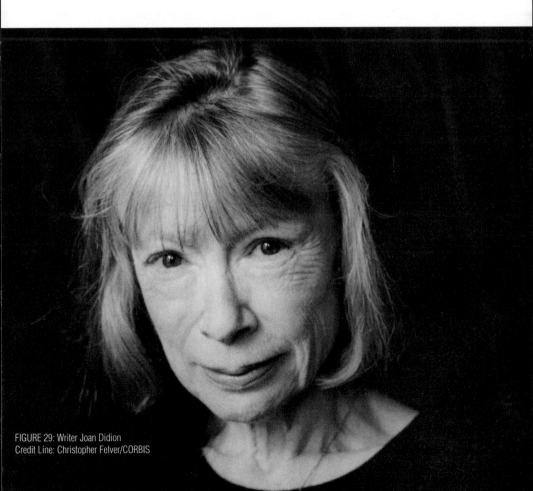

FIGURE 29: Writer Joan Didion
Credit Line: Christopher Felver/CORBIS

CLUSTER HEADACHES

The Classification Committee of the International Headache Society has described cluster headaches as "attacks of severe, strictly unilateral pain, orbitally, supraorbitally and/or temporally, lasting 15 to 180 minutes and occurring from once every other day to eight times a day."[1] These headaches have been called ciliary or migrainous neuralgia, histaminic cephalalgia, Vidian and Sluder's neuralgia, and Horton's headache. E. Charles Kunkle labeled this condition "cluster headache," referring to the periodicity of these headaches that occur in series or "cluster periods."

The etiology of cluster headache is unknown. During acute cluster attacks, extracranial vasodilation and increased cerebral blood flow occur, and the nucleus of the trigeminal nerve descending to the C2 segment becomes hyperactive unilaterally. The internal carotid artery and its proximal branches are recognized as the main peripheral source of the pain.

Three major events are involved in cluster headache: the cluster period, triggering of the attack, and pain production. Certain metabolic and clinical alterations occur during the cluster series. At the onset of a cluster series, an increase in levels of histamine and serotonin occur, and decrease dramatically at the end of a cluster period. Although the provocateur for a series is unknown, during a series, alcohol is a well-recognized trigger of the acute attacks. Researchers have evoked a cluster attack using sublingual nitroglycerin or histamine injected subcutaneously. Cluster headache patients also decrease or stop smoking during a series, as the intensity and duration of the acute attacks appear to be affected by this habit.

OUTWARDLY, I WAS A CALM PRODUCER-DIRECTOR; INWARDLY, A VAT OF SEETHING SOUR WINE. SOMETHING HAD TO BLOW. IT BLEW ON NEW YEAR'S EVE. PAPER HATS ASKEW, WE WERE CAROLING THE BIRTH OF 1961 IN THE LA QUINTA HOTEL DINING ROOM, WHEN SUDDENLY — A HUGE PHANTOM BIRD SANK THREE TALONS OF ITS ANGRY CLAW DEEP INTO MY HEAD AND FACE, AND TRIED TO LIFT ME. NO WARNINGS, NO PRELIMINARY SIGNS. JUST WHAM! A MASSIVE, KILLING PAIN OVER MY RIGHT EYE. LEAVING, LU, JIM AND MARION, FRANK AND PRISCILLA TO FROLIC IT UP, I CLUTCHED MY HEAD STUMBLED OUT TO THE BROAD LAWNS, AND SKULKED ALONG OLEANDER HEDGES TO THE DESERTED TENNIS COURTS. AND THERE IN THE DARKNESS, I MOANED, PANTED, BALLOONED MY CHEEKS, BLEW OUT SHORT BURSTS OF AIR, LICKED HOT LIPS, WIPED TEARS THAT POURED OUT OF MY RIGHT EYE, AND CLAWED AT MY HEAD, TRYING TO UPROOT THE FIENDISH TALONS FROM THEIR IRON GRIP. ONE RACKING HOUR LATER, THE TALONS LET GO. THE PAROXYSM EASED AS SUDDENLY AS IT HAD CONVULSED. EUPHORIA SET IN. LU AND FRANK, JR., FOUND ME CHUCKLING TO MYSELF, "IT'S GONE, DARLING! A WHOPPING HEADACHE. BUT IT'S GONE."[51]

— *Frank Capra*

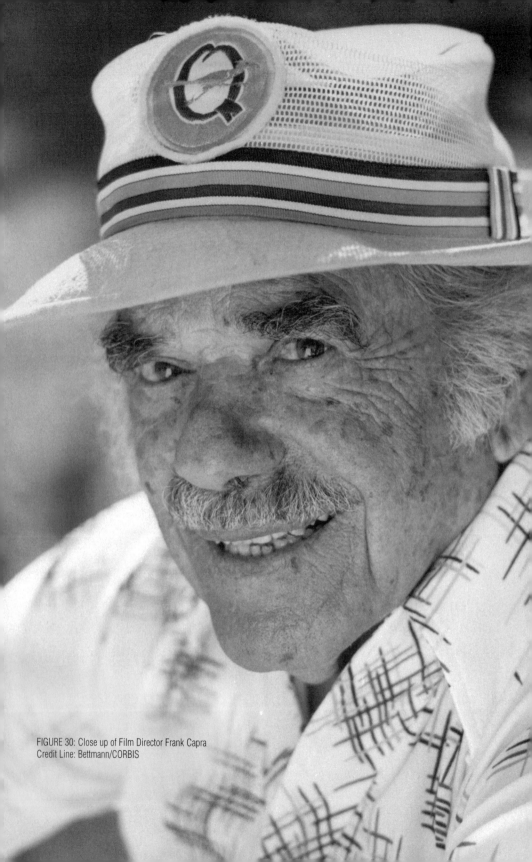

FIGURE 30: Close up of Film Director Frank Capra
Credit Line: Bettmann/CORBIS

It would be impossible to improve on the description of an acute cluster headache attack by Frank Capra (1897 to 1991), the great film director. At age 63, without warning Capra suffered his first cluster headache. An Italian immigrant who had known poverty in both his native Sicily and later his new home of California, he had made a tremendous success of himself. Although he received a degree in chemical engineering from Cal Tech in 1918, Capra struggled to find employment after leaving the Army. By chance, and to the viewing public's fortune, Capra found his way into the movie industry. His films have epitomized the indomitability of the human spirit — *It Happened One Night, Mr. Deeds Goes to Town, Lost Horizon, Mr. Smith Goes to Washington, Meet John Doe, It's A Wonderful Life*. His success in films and in life had prevailed but now, on December 31, 1960, Capra would know the pain of cluster headaches.

Cluster headaches are typified by the brief duration of the acute attacks, lasting from 10 minutes to 3 hours. The pain is always unilateral, remaining on one side of the head during the entire series. Many cluster patients will complain of localized pain around or behind one eye. The pain has been described as stabbing, boring, or sharp knifelike sensations in the eye, and of such severity that patients have contemplated suicide during a series.

The defining characteristic of cluster headaches is the occurrence in a series — ranging from a few weeks to 3 or 4 months. During a series, the headache may occur several times per day, usually waking the patient at the same time each night. Frank Capra learned the routine of this malady:

TWO MORE ATTACKS THAT NIGHT LEFT GROVELING ON THE FLOOR. IN THE MORNING, I CALLED OUR DOCTOR FRIEND STANLEY IMERMAN. THREE DIFFERENT NEUROLOGISTS EXAMINED ME; TUNING, THUMPING; X RAYS OF THE HEAD; ENCEPHALOGRAMS OF THE BRAIN WAVES. ALL NORMAL. THE AGONIZING ATTACKS CONTINUED NIGHTLY — TWO, THREE, FOUR. THERE IS NO KNOWN CURE FOR "CLUSTER" HEADACHES, SAID THE EXPERTS, AND STRONGLY ADVISED CALLING OFF POCKETFUL. ONE NEUROLOGIST SUGGESTED A POSSIBLE PALLIATIVE. HORTON'S TREATMENT WAS ROUGH. IT CONSISTED OF A SMALL INJECTION OF SODIUM PHOSPHATE, THE DOSE DOUBLING EVERY DAY FOR SOME TEN DAYS. I WOULD TRY ANYTHING.

In contrast to the patient experiencing an acute migraine attack who will recline in a dark, quiet room, the patient enduring a cluster episode prefers to be upright and walking about the room:

THAT NIGHT THE HEADACHES RETURNED. ONE EACH NIGHT, THEN TWO, THREE, FOUR. I CLIMBED THE WALLS. ONE HOUR OF EXCRUCIATING AGONY, THEN SOME FITFUL, ONLY TO WAKE UP SCREAMING WITH PAIN.

Associated symptoms include lacrimation, nasal congestion or rhinorrhea, facial flushing, partial Horner's syndrome, conjunctival injection, and ptosis of the ipsilateral eyelid.

These headaches are more frequent in the spring and fall. Ninety percent of cluster headache sufferers are male, and will note the first occurrence of these headaches during their twenties or thirties. Frank Capra did not fit the pattern — his first cluster series occurred when he was 63. When his headaches reappeared in 1962, Capra consulted Doctor Arnold Friedman at Montefiore Hospital in New York City. Doctor Friedman advised Capra: *"Because," he explained, "in their active stage they come in clusters, like grapes. We know very little about them, and less about how to treat them. But men over fifty-five very rarely suffer them. You must be some kind of a specimen."*

The cluster series is self-limiting, usually continuing for a few weeks to several months. For Frank Capra, he notes that his clusters went into a "passive stage" in the fall of 1963. However, he never again directed a film for mass audiences and limited himself to documentaries, and the producing of his autobiography in 1971.

For some unfortunate patients, the cluster headaches do not abate, and the individual will not experience a remission of these headaches for intervals lasting longer than 14 days. This condition, chronic cluster headaches, is difficult to manage.

CLUSTER VARIANTS

Other forms of cluster headache have been identified, including chronic paroxysmal hemicrania and cluster headache variant. These headaches are also known as indomethacin responsive headaches. Chronic paroxysmal hemicrania (CPH) is characterized by the excessive daily frequency of the attacks, described as jabs, occurring 15 or more times per day. Patients describe the severity as intense, and identify certain movements, such as bending the head forward, as headache triggers. CPH is a rarely documented disorder, and its dramatic response to indomethacin is highly characteristic.

The prevalence of cluster headache variant is much higher.[52] Three types of pain are linked to cluster headache variant, and may occur in any combination with these patients: atypical cluster headache (atypical location, duration, and frequency); multiple jabs lasting only a few seconds and occurring several times per day, which can be triggered by certain head movements; and background vascular headaches that are continuous, usually sharply localized and often unilateral, which can vary in severity and may be throbbing or exacerbated during exercise. These headaches are also highly responsive to indomethacin. For those patients refractory to indomethacin, the antidepressants, propranolol, or lithium may be considered.

TENSION-TYPE HEADACHES

ADRIAN HAD NOT ASKED FOR A PHYSICIAN, BECAUSE HE WANTED
TO INTERPRET HIS SUFFERINGS AS FAMILIAR AND HEREDITARY,
AS MERELY AN ACUTE INTENSIFICATION OF HIS FATHER'S MIGRAINE.
IT WAS FRAU SCHWEIGESTILL WHO AT LAST INSISTED ON CALLING
IN DR. KÜRBIS, THE WALDSHUT DISTRICT PHYSICIAN, THE SAME
WHO HAD ONCE DELIVERED THE FRÄULEIN FROM BAYREUTH.
THE GOOD MAN WOULD NOT HEAR OF MIGRAINE, SINCE THE
OFTEN EXCESSIVE PAINS WERE NOT ONE-SIDED AS IS THE CASE
WITH MIGRAINE BUT CONSISTED IN A RAGING TORMENT IN AND
ABOVE BOTH EYES, AND MOREOVER WERE CONSIDERED BY THE
PHYSICIAN TO BE A SECONDARY SYMPTOM.

– *Doctor Faustus, Thomas Mann,* 1947

Thomas Mann (1875 to 1955) is considered the leading German writer of the early part of the last century and possibly a migraine sufferer. His literary career started with contributors to *Simplicissimus*, a literary satirical journal, and eventually became a free-lance writer while living in Italy (1895 to 1897).

During his exile from his beloved Munich, Mann wrote *Doktor Faustus*, which contains his description of migraine. In his rendition of the classic tale, Mann presents Adrian Leverkuhn as a composer who makes a pact with the devil in order to achieve an artistic breakthrough to creative vitality. The physician who examines Adrian rules out migraine as the cause of the composer's headaches due to its occurrence on both sides of the head. As Mann notes, migraine is usually a one-sided headache. However, it can occur bilaterally, primarily affecting the frontal area of the head, often surrounding the eyes. The fictional Doctor Kürbis wisely considered the headaches as a secondary symptom — headache is not the disorder but rather a manifestation of a problem.

Tension-type (muscle contraction) headaches are considered a manifestation of the body's response to stress, anxiety, depression, emotional conflicts, fatigue, and repressed hostility. Two types of tension-type headache have been identified, episodic and chronic. Episodic tension-type headache has been experienced by most individuals over a lifetime. The pain is recurrent, lasting from minutes to days, and can be described as pressure or a tightening sensation. The headaches are usually mild to moderate and easily managed with OTC analgesics, including the NSAIDS and acetaminophen. Patients experiencing episodic tension-type headaches will rarely consult a physician. In contrast to migraine, these headaches are bilateral and are not associated with other complaints, such as nausea and vomiting.

The frequency of the chronic tension-type headaches are the distinguishing characteristic, usually occurring on a daily or almost daily basis. The headaches are usually continuous, and may have a diurnal variation to the severity. Typically, the

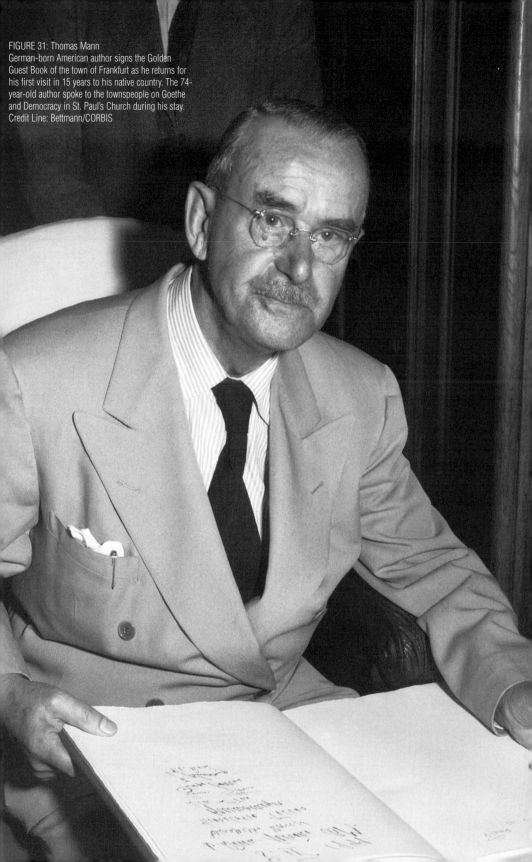

headaches are mild to moderate, and can be described as viselike ache, pressure sensations, bandlike sensations around the head, soreness, drawing, or a weight. The pain is bilateral, usually located in the forehead, temples, and back of the head or neck. Pain may radiate to the neck or the shoulders. Sharply localized nodules may be observed on palpation.

IN THE BURROWS OF THE NIGHTMARE
WHERE THE JUSTICE NAKED IS.
TIMES WATCHES FROM THE SHADOW
AND COUGHS WHEN YOU WOULD KISS.
IN HEADACHES AND IN WORRY
VAGUELY LIFE LEAKS AWAY
AND TIME WILL HAVE HIS FANCY
TOMORROW OR TODAY.

— From Birthday Poem, W. H. Auden

Wystan Hugh Auden (1907 to 1973) was a British-born poet who became a U.S. citizen in 1946. He is regarded as one of the most important poets of the 20th century. Auden was educated at Oxford, and gained recognition as a member of socialist writers, including Stephen Spender and Christopher Isherwood. With Isherwood, Auden wrote three plays, including *The Dog Beneath the Skin*. Throughout Auden's poems, one of the prominent themes is the dissolution of civilization and culture.

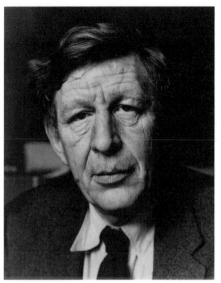

FIGURE 32: Poet W.H. Auden
Credit Line: CORBIS

In his brief allusion to headaches, Auden indicates that headaches do impact on life — letting life "leak away." The pain suffered throughout life is inevitable, and you should learn to live with it — a stratagem often recommended by physicians who are at a loss when dealing with chronic pain. This pessimistic view can be counteracted with education of physicians as well as their patients and the families so affected by this chronic disorder.

During the initial interview, the examining physician should question the patient about family, marital, work, and social relationships. The psychological inventory should include questions about life stresses, occupation, habits, personality traits, sexual problems, and methods of coping with stress. Patients may appear extremely distressed or depressed, and appear to lack emotion. Spontaneous crying may also occur.

TENSION-TYPE HEADACHES

*SHE ALMOST PLOTTED SOME SCHEME OF A HEADACHE, IN WHICH
SHE MIGHT BE ENABLE NOT TO SHOW HERSELF TILL AFTER DINNER.
'I AM SO BLIND THAT I CAN HARDLY SEE OUT OF MY EYES,'
SHE SAID TO THE MAID, ACTUALLY BEGINNING THE SCHEME.*

— Phineas Redux, Anthony Trollope, 1874

Anthony Trollope (1815 to 1882) was a prolific novelist in Victorian England. He delighted his readers with social satires and romantic stories. Our contemporary critics consider the use of mild irony in Trollope's works as an instrument to discuss serious moral issues.

In clinical practice, too often we observe chronic headache sufferers using their headaches to avoid responsibilities, such as missing school or work, avoiding a trip or social event. Other headache sufferers may use the headaches to gain attention — from parents, spouses, children, or significant others. If these scenarios are obvious, the physician treating the patient must involve the family and other interested parties into the therapeutic approach — to promote healthy behavior by positive reinforcement. In other words, when the patient is healthy (headache-free), attention is given to the individual so that the "well-behavior" is reinforced. This method of pain management was established by Wilbur Fordyce at the University of Washington in Seattle. The Seattle model of pain is based on the increasing complexity of adapting to pain, from the introduction of the pain triggers or stimuli, to the suffering, and finally to pain behavior.

In observing pain behavior, the physicians and other health care providers will note that the patient has certain expectations about the pain and about how others will react to the pain problem. Breaking that pattern of behavior is the mission of specialized treatment units for chronic pain. We must encourage the pain sufferer to cast away the shadows of a victim and aim at pain remission.

The patient with chronic tension-type headaches due to anxiety will complain of an annoying headache not associated with other symptoms. Typically, these patients will note a difficulty falling asleep, a feature that distinguished these headaches from those due to depression.

Patients with chronic tension-type headaches due to depression will describe morning as the worst time of day. These patients experience early or frequent awakening, and may complain of a variety of physical symptoms, such as shortness of breath, constipation, weight loss, fatigue, decreased libido, palpations, and menstrual changes. Psychic complaints include poor concentration, low or no ambition, indecisiveness, poor memory, loss of interest, and suicidal ideation. The emotional complaints often voiced by these patients involve feelings of hopelessness, guilt, unworthiness, as well as fear of insanity, physical disease, or death. Some patients will ruminate over the past, present, and future. Commonly, the patient will identify a particular event as triggering the headaches, such as the death of a loved one, an accident, or surgery. The event may be perceived as more serious and disproportionate to the actual occurrence.

HEADACHE TREATMENT —
A HISTORICAL PERSPECTIVE

The "Blister" was one form of therapy which was touted for a number of disorders, including epilepsy and other neurological conditions. Although not as drastic as trepanning, the blister was very painful. The procedure was clearly delineated in the text, *Bibliotheca Anatomica, Medica, Chirurgica, Etc*, published in London, in 1712.[53] The agent used was "a medicament prepared from *Cantharides* or Spanish Flies, which being laid on the Skin, by its crimony raises Blisters or Bladders." The agent, *Cantharis vesicatoria*, is also known as the "blister beetle." The author of this prescription was Pierre Dionis, listed in the volume as the "Chief Surgeon to the Present Dauphiness." The flies were to be dried and powdered, and mixed with "Leaven and Vinegar," and the solution was to remain on the skin for at least 4 or 5 hours, an interval considered sufficient for adequate size blisters to develop. After this time period, the blisters were lanced, in order to set the "serous Humour" to be emitted. If the original problem continued, the blisters may be left for 2 or 3 days, and "the more the Patient is eased."[54]

William Heberden, published a classic description of headache in his text, *Commentaries on the History and Cure of Diseases.* He notes that:

"THE NATURE OF HEAD -ACHS IS EXTREMELY OBSCURE.
THEIR MANIFEST CAUSES ARE VERY VARIOUS, AND OFTEN
CONTRARY TO ONE ANOTHER. THEY PROBABLY THEREFORE
ARISE FROM DIFFERENT DISORDERS."

Heberden observed that severe, recurring headaches are usually not fatal, and he notes philosophically, that *"It is some consolation for a man to know, that if he cannot cure his distemper, he will however have a good chance to outlive it."* Heberden describes migraine with aura (classic migraine) as "hemicrania." He also depicts the associated gastrointestinal symptoms of acute migraine attacks.

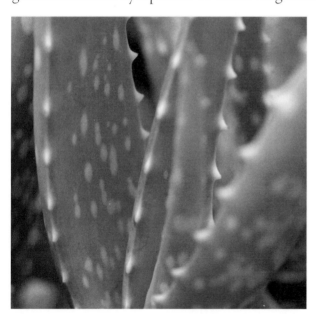

Heberden's recommendations for treatment include some general measures — avoidance of noise, crowds, anxiety, and fatigue; rest, quiet, warmth, and fresh air are beneficial. He advised the reader:

FIGURE 33: Aloe Vera Plant Close Up. Credit Line: FOODPIX

"THOUGH EVERY KNOWN REMEDY FOR HEAD-ACHS HAS AT TIMES FAILED, YET AMONG THOSE WHICH HAVE SELDOMEST DISAPPOINTED MY EXPECTATIONS, I FIND A PERPETUAL BLISTER TO THE HEAD, THE TAKING AWAY OF SIX OUNCES OF BLOOD BY CUPPING UPON THE SHOULDERS ONCE IN SIX WEEKS, AND PILLS MADE OF ONE GRAIN OF ALOËS AND EITHER FOUR GRAINS OF COLUMBO ROOT, OR HALF A SCRUPTLE OF PULV. MYRRH. COMP. TAKEN EVERY NIGHT. EMETICS ARE OFTEN HIGHLY SERVICEABLE; THE STRAIN TO VOMIT AGGRAVATES THE PAIN MUCH LESS THAN MIGHT BE FEARED, AND THEY HAVE BEEN REPEATED EVERY MONTH WITH SUCCESS; NOR IS IT UNUSUAL FOR A SPONTANEOUS VOMITING TO CURE A HEADACH. THE PAIN OF THE HEAD SO COMMON IN THE BEGINNING OF FEVERS IS MUCH RELIEVED BY IT; BUT FOR THIS PARTICULAR HEAD-ACH A BLISTER BETWEEN THE SHOULDERS MAY BE RECOMMENDED AS A SPECIFIC. WARM FOMENTATIONS OF THE HEAD, OR FEET, OFTEN GIVE PRESENT EASE; AND TINCTURE OPII HAS BE USEFUL FOR THE SAME PURPOSE."

The aloes described by Doctor Heberden are the dried juice of the leaves of *Aloe*, a large genus of liliaceous plants. Aloe (Mauritus hemp) is an agave plant, native to Brazil. Despite its name, it is not a true hemp. Aloe was introduced into Mauritus (in the Indian ocean off Madagascar) in the late 18th century. The fiber is made into bagging and sometimes mixed with other fibers for rope. The "columbo root," the ingredient to be combined with the aloes, may be either the African calumba root (*Jateorhiza columba*) or the East Indian columba wood (*Coscinium fenestratum*) — both contain the extremely bitter substance called columbin. The myrrh is an equally bitter resin, derived chiefly from the *Courmiphora abyssinica*, a tree found in Africa and Arabia.

Reverend Edward Stone, from Chipping Norton, Oxfordshire, in England, is usually recognized as providing the first scientific description of the beneficial effects of willow bark. In a letter (1763) to the Earl of Macclesfield, he describes successfully treating patients with fever (usually related to malaria) with 20 grains of powdered willow bark in a dram of water every 4 hours.[55] Stone related:

> AS THIS TREE DELIGHTS IN A MOIST OR WET SOIL,
> WHERE AGUES CHIEFLY ABOUND, THE GENERAL MAXIM THAT
> MANY NATURAL MALADIES CARRY THEIR CURES ALONG WITH
> THEM OR THAT THEIR REMEDIES LIE NOT FAR FROM THEIR CAUSES
> WAS SO VERY APPOSITE TO THIS PARTICULAR CASE THAT I COULD
> NOT HELP APPLYING IT; AND THAT THIS MIGHT BE THE
> INTENTION OF PROVIDENCE HERE, I MUST OWN, HAD SOME
> LITTLE WEIGHT WITH ME.

Continental blockage imposed by Napoleon at the beginning of the 19th century, in order to destroy British trade, made the supply of Peruvian bark a much sought-after commodity.

Descriptions of headache and headache treatment abound during this century. John Fordyce published *De Hemicrania* in 1758.[56] Fordyce, a migraine sufferer himself, provided a series of clinical observations based largely on his own headache condition. He noted that his left side was more frequently affected than his right side, and that he experienced a premonitory depression before an attack. During the attack, he noted increased urinary output. Fordyce also noted the relationship between migraine and menstruation. His preferred remedy was *Valeriana sylvestris* which "actually relieved greatly and cured me when I had for four years suffered so much oppression that I almost grew weary of life."

In *De Hemicrania Menstrua*, Fordyce detailed the relationship of ovarian activity upon migraine. He described his management of the particularly severe headaches in the Marquise of Brandenburg.

Another migraine sufferer, John Fothergill (1712 to 1780) also published reports of his headache condition. In 1778, he described migraine as "a disease which, though it occurs very frequently, has not yet obtained a place in the systematic catalogues." Fothergill was particularly interested in the dietary triggers of headache, and was probably the first to identify chocolate as a headache precipitant. He did not approve of the diet habits of his contemporaries in England. He felt that more people suffered from immoderate eating than by hard drinking. He recalled a discussion with the famous Doctor Mandeville when dining with the Earl of Macclesfield:

"DOCTOR, IS THIS WHOLESOME?"

"DOES YOUR LORDSHIP LIKE IT?"

"YES"

"DOES IT AGREE WITH YOUR LORDSHIP?"

"YES"

"WHY THEN IT IS WHOLESOME."

Fothergill also described the use of coffee, and the emergence of coffee houses in London. Coffee, which had been brought to Europe from Turkey in the middle of the 17th century, had become very popular to the point that duties and licenses were imposed on the coffeehouses. Charles II, in 1675, tried to close the coffee houses, describing them as "Seminaries of Sedition."

In 1652, it was reported that Otto Tackenius of Venice used a compound of a volatile salt of vipers and an extract of steel to cured "hundreds of headaches deemed incurable."[55]

For migraine prophylaxis, many practitioners recommended cures associated with the gastrointestinal symptoms of migraine. Abernethy (1764 to 1831) promulgated the practice of ritual purgation for the treatment of a variety of disorders, including migraine. Calomel was often used, and later a preparation — a combination of soap with aloes — was used with occasional additions of nux vornica. Regular purgation was recommended well into the 20th century. Vegetable bitters were suggested by Tissot, in 1790, for migraine sufferers with gastric atony.

Fordyce and other early physicians associated migraine with gout.[53] Simple diets have been recommended for centuries. Buzzard (1831 to 1919) suggested an oleaginous diet, consuming cod liver oil to prevent the migraine. Fordyce, however, felt that hot buttered toast could trigger an acute episode. Liveing also noted that "I have known instances where abstinence from butter for a term reduced the number of attacks — such are the caprices of this singular disease."[57]

J. Addington Symonds in 1858, presented three Goulstonian lectures to the Royal College of Physicians on the topic of migraine. He recommended a daily tumblerful of salty water one hour before breakfast.[58] Haller reportedly abated his headaches by drinking large amounts of water and by simplifying his diet.

In the 19th century, migraine sufferers were advised to avoid excessive intellectual strain. If unavoidable, remedies such as henbane (hyoscyamus) or bromide of potassium were to be considered. Osler, in 1916, noted that excessive book-work would impact on the headaches of children:

"ON NO ACCOUNT SHOULD MIGRAINOUS CHILDREN
BE ALLOWED IN SCHOOL TO COMPETE FOR PRIZES." [59]

Emotional stress was a long-identified headache trigger. The bromides and henbane, as well as zinc and valerian, used singly or in combination, were recommended for these attacks precipitated by emotional upheaval.

Although it was recognized as a headache provocateur, physical exercise was recommended for some migraine sufferers. Carolus Linnaeus (1707 to 1778), the Swedish botanist, is noted for developing the classification system for plants, animals, and microorganisms. He is also a noted migraine sufferer. It has been reported that Linnaeus experienced visual hallucinations as part of his aura — he would often seen visions of himself prior to the onset of an acute headache. In one anecdote, Linnaeus entered a class that he was about to teach. Seeing the vision of himself in the room, he said, "Oh, I'm there already," and closed the door. Linnaeus reportedly claimed that he cured his migraine by taking exercise every day before dinner.

FIGURE 34: Coffee Plant. Credit Line: BOTANICA

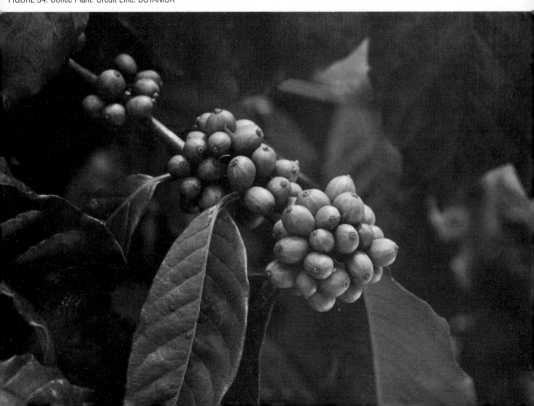

Liveing noted that "exercise must be proportioned at first to the strength and habits of the individual and any sudden strain should be, as far as possible, avoided." Liveing's philosophy was that a well-regulated mode of life would prevent these headaches — "establish a rigorous uniformity of life, to make on day the exact counterpart of another, and to avoid irregularities of every kind."

For a migraine sufferer in mid-19th century who was fortunate to find a physician to treat the condition, a number of agents were used. Robert Bently Todd, in 1858, recommended potassium iodide. Osler suggested that cannabis indica was probably the most satisfactory. Gowers prescribed trinitrotoluene, an essential ingredient of the well-known Gower's mixture, which was still being used in the 1940s. This treatment was a combination of liquid trinitrin m. I, liquid strychnine m III, tincture of gelsemia m XV, phenazone gr. V, sodil bromide gr XV, ac. Hydrobrom dil. M. X, aq chloroform ad drams I. This preparation was to be used three times daily.

Liveing's favored remedy was a combination of belladonna and henbane. Patent medicines were very popular, such as Becquerel's pills consisting of quinine sulphate, extract of digitalis, and extract of colchicum. Debt's pills were a similar preparation.

Caffeine to this day is used in migraine treatment. Guarana (Brazilian cocoa) was used during the 19th century.

It was prepared from the seeds of an Amazonian climbing plant of the soapberry variety (*paulinne cupana or sorbilis*). This concoction contained 3 to 5 times as much caffeine as ordinary coffee beans. Gowers felt that caffeine did not live up to its expectations as an effective migraine treatment.

Identifying and avoiding headache triggers can be a first step in prevention. Because migraine patients are particularly sensitive, a regular sleep and meal schedule should be maintained. Although stress cannot be avoided, instruction of coping strategies may be very beneficial to migraine patients.

Nondrug measures can be instituted for migraine patients. The application of an ice bag or a commercial cold-pack to the affected area may provide some relief. One of the major figures of the U.S. Civil War was the best known of the Union commanders Ulysses S. Grant (1822 to 1885), who later served as 18th president of the United States. Unlike Thomas Jefferson, Grant did not leave extensive journals nor correspondence. He did maintain a wartime journal, as did many of his colleagues. George Meade, his second-in-command, recalled Grant riding into camp on the evening of April 8, 1865: "(Grant) *had one of his sick headaches, which are rare, but cause him fearful pain, such as almost overcomes his iron stoicism.*" His journal entry for that date truly give testimony to his migraine problem:

HEADACHE TREATMENT — A HISTORICAL PERSPECTIVE

❧

"I WAS SUFFERING VERY SEVERELY WITH A SICK HEADACHE,
AND STOPPED AT A FARM HOUSE ON THE ROAD SOME DISTANCE
TO THE REAR OF THE MAIN BODY OF THE ARMY. I SPENT THE NIGHT
IN BATHING MY FEET IN HOT WATER AND MUSTARD, AND PUTTING
MUSTARD PLASTERS ON MY WRISTS AND THE BACK PART OF MY NECK,
HOPING TO BE CURED BY MORNING."[60]

❧

Unfortunately, the headache remained when the general awakened. Soon after he arose, a messenger arrived with a communication from General Robert E. Lee. On the previous day, Lee had refused to surrender but now indicated that he was willing to talk peace terms. Grant's next journal entry reports:

❧

"WHEN THE OFFICER REACHED ME, I WAS STILL SUFFERING
FROM THE SICK HEADACHE; BUT THE INSTANT I SAW THE
CONTENTS OF THE NOTE I WAS CURED."

❧

Grant later commented to his aide, Colonel Horace Porter that:

❧

"THE PAIN IN MY HEAD SEEMED TO LEAVE ME THE
MOMENT I GOT LEE'S LETTER."

❧

Although mustard plasters are not a popular remedy for migraine attacks, relief of stress — provided to General Grant by General Lee's surrender — would be highly recommended for any migraine sufferer.

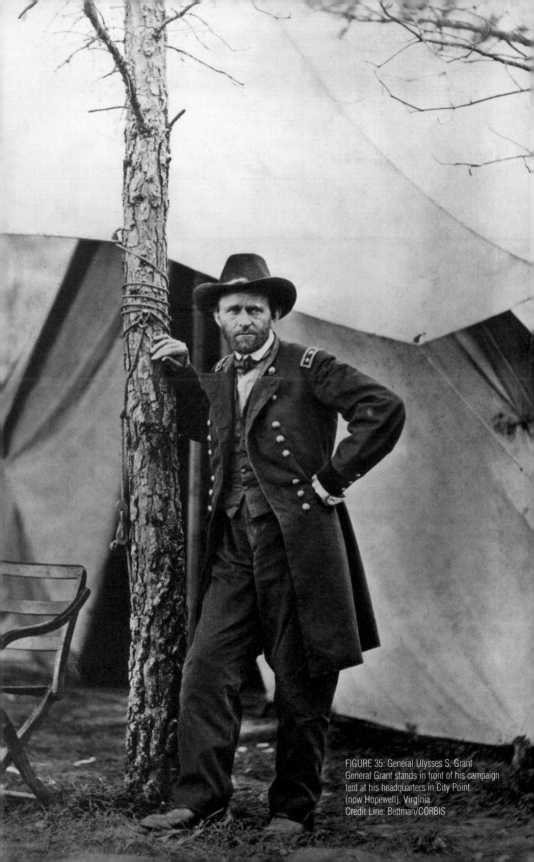

FIGURE 35: General Ulysses S. Grant
General Grant stands in front of his campaign
tent at his headquarters in City Point
(now Hopewell), Virginia.
Credit Line: Bettman/CORBIS

CONCLUSION

"WELL, MY DEAR MISS SARTI, AND HOW DO YOU FEEL NOW? —
A LITTLE BETTER, I SEE. I THOUGHT YOU WOULD BE, SITTING QUIETLY
HERE. THESE HEADACHES, NOW, ARE ALL FROM WEAKNESS. YOU MUST
NOT OVEREXERT YOURSELF, AND YOU MUST TAKE BITTERS. I USED TO
HAVE JUST THE SAME SORT OF HEADACHES WHEN I WAS YOUR AGE,
AND OLD DR. SAMSON USED TO SAY TO MY MOTHER, MADAM, WHAT
YOUR DAUGHTER SUFFERS FROM IS WEAKNESS."

— Scenes of Clerical Life, George Eliot, 1858

George Eliot is the pseudonym of British novelist, Mary Anne Evans (1819 to 1880). Although she is not usually included on the list of famous migraineurs, the above description of headache hints at some form of personal knowledge of this malady. Eliot's description of Lady Cheverel's reaction to headache is all too true, whether in 19th century drawing rooms or 21st century emergency departments. Because we have no physical measure of headache, headache is often dismissed

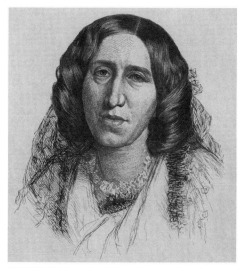

FIGURE 36: Etching by Paul Adolphe Rajon After George Eliot by Frederick William Burton. This etching was done after the original portrait in the National Portrait Gallery, London, by Frederick William Burton.
Credit Line: Bettman/CORBIS

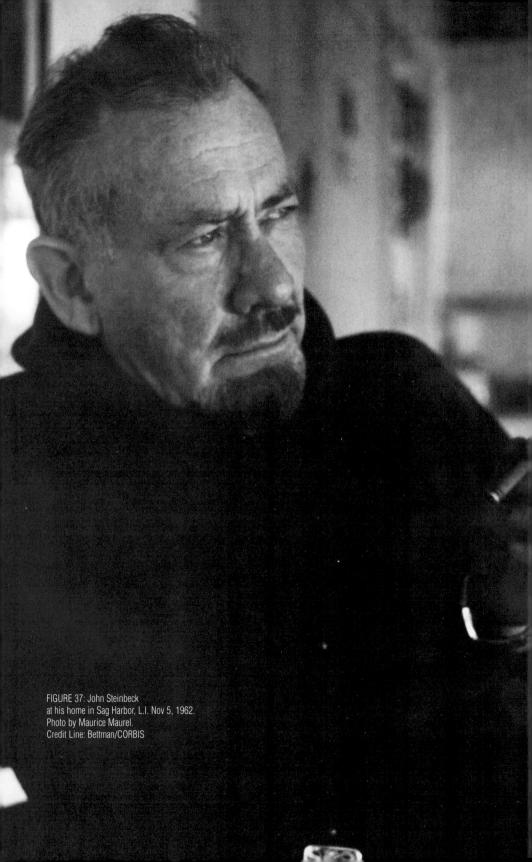

FIGURE 37: John Steinbeck
at his home in Sag Harbor, L.I. Nov 5, 1962.
Photo by Maurice Maurel.
Credit Line: Bettman/CORBIS

as not real, as a weakness. Our remedy for this interpretation of pain is public education and continuing studies on the impact of headache on society, the economy, and the individual's quality of life.

❧

HER HUSBAND KNEW HER HEADACHES, AND THEY WERE DREADFUL. THEY TWISTED HER FACE AND REDUCED HER TO A PANTING, SWEATING, GRINNING, QUIVERING BLOB OF PAIN. THEY FILLED A ROOM AND A HOUSE. THEY GOT INTO EVERYONE AROUND HER. MR. PRITCHARD USUALLY CAME WHEN SHE WAS NERVOUS AND WHEN THINGS, THROUGH NO FAULT OF HER OWN, WERE NOT GOING WELL.

❧

— *The Wayward Bus, John Steinbeck, 1947*

John Steinbeck (1902 to 1968), a Nobel prize winner in literature, is known for his stories about the downtrodden, such as the Joad family in *The Grapes of Wrath*. The description of the migraine sufferer in *The Wayward Bus*, Mrs. Pritchard not only provides a thorough characterization of an acute attack, but it also hints at the impact of her pain to her family. Steinbeck further alludes to the prejudice faced by chronic headache sufferers. Mrs. Pritchard details how she is accused of malingering by her unfeeling daughter:

❧

THEY SEEMED TO BE SELFISH, THESE HEADACHES, AND YET THEY WERE NOT. THE PAIN WAS REAL. NO ONE COULD SIMULATE SUCH AGONIZING PAIN. MRS. PRITCHARD DREADED THEM MORE THAN ANYTHING IN THE WORLD. A GOOD ONE COULD MAKE THE WHOLE HOUSE VIBRATE WITH HORROR.

❧

Mrs. Pritchard, and her family, were unwilling victims of the very real migraine attacks. Steinbeck's narration could be used for any form of public education platform on chronic headaches. Did Steinbeck suffer from headaches? If not, he did then understand how headache changes an individual and can become a focus of a family's life, whether the victim is the parent or the child. Mrs. Pritchard's daughter dismissed the pain as "psychosomatic" but Steinbeck knew better. He understood that the pain could be triggered by anxiety and stress but the symptoms were all too real.

To conclude this text, we must look back on the writer first quoted in this book, George Bernard Shaw. Shaw showed early signs of the precociousness observed so frequently in our famous headache sufferers. He treated most everyone in the same ill manner he used with Nansen — one biographer notes that Shaw was condescending to his governess. At age 25, he contracted a mild form of smallpox. This problem left his face pockmarked, and he suffered psychologically. Shaw remained a vegetarian all of his adult life, believing foods to be a trigger for all sorts of complaints.

In 1898, Shaw at age 42, described himself as:

❧

I HAVE BEEN DINNING INTO THE PUBLIC HEAD THAT I AM AN
EXTRAORDINARILY WITTY, BRILLIANT AND CLEVER MAN.
THAT IS NOW PART OF THE PUBLIC OPINION OF ENGLAND; AND NO
POWER IN HEAVEN OR ON EARTH WILL EVER CHANGE IT.

❧

Shaw's obsession with perfection reflects the migraine personality. His confrontation with Nansen may certainly remind us of one of his most famous quotes — used at the funeral of Senator Robert F. Kennedy:

YOU SEE THINGS AND SAY "WHY?" BUT I DREAM THINGS THAT NEVER WERE, AND I SAY "WHY NOT?"

Perhaps, we should follow this directive when we consider the complaint of headache. We can wonder why the headache is there, but we should also seek to end this terrible complaint.

REFERENCE

1. Pearson H. *Bernard Shaw*. London: Collins; 1942; 242-243.

2. Jack DB. One hundred years of aspirin. *Lancet*. 1997; 350:437-439.

3. *Colossians* 4:14.

4. Caldwell T. *Dear and Glorious Physician*. New York: Doubleday; 1959.

5. Preuss J. *Biblical and Talmudic Medicine* (Rosner F, translator and editor). New York: Sanhedrin Press; 1978.

6. Shabbath 11a

7. Rosner F. Headache in the writings of Moses Maimonides and other Hebrew sages. *Headache*. 1993; 33:315-319.

8. Chullin 105b

9. Nedarim 49b

10. Proverbs 1:9.

11. I Chronicles 4:10.

12. Nedarim 41a.

13. Horton BT. Note on a biblical headache. *JAMA*. 1975; 234:1019. (Letter)

14. Kings II 4:18-20.

15. Rosner F. A Biblical headache. *JAMA*. 1976; 235:1327. (Letter)

16. Bollet AJ. A case history from the Bible. *Resident Staff Physician*. 1979; 39.

17. Rosner F. *Headache* 1993; 33:315-319.

18. Rosner F. *The Medical Aphorisms of Moses Maimonides*. Haifa, Israel: Maimonides Research Institute; 1989; 111.

19. Muntner S. *The Medical Writings of Moses Maimonides*. Treatise on Asthma. Philadelphia: Lippincott; 1963.

20. Rosner F. *Medicine in the Mishneh Torah of Maimonides*. New York: CDEV; 1984; 156.

21. Islet H, Hasenfratz H, O'Neill T. A sixth-century Irish headache cure and its use in a South German monastery. *Cephalalgia*. 1996; 16:536-540.

22. Friedman AF. The headache in history, literature, and legend. *Bull NY Acad Med*. 1972; 48:661-681.

23. Magnus HF. *Superstitions in Medicine*. New York: Funk & Wagnalls; 1908.

24. Fox M. *Illuminations of Hildegard of Bingen*. Santa Fe, New Mexico: Bear & Company; 1985.

25. Unlein G. *Meditations with Hildegard of Bingen*. Santa Fe, New Mexico: Bear & Company; 1982.

26. Quoted by Wilson SAR, Bruce AN. *Neurology*, 2nd edition. Baltimore: Williams and Wilkins; 1955, volume 3, p 1704.

27. Singer C. The visions of Hildegard of Bingen. *From Magic to Science: Essays on the Scientific Twilight*. New York: Dover Publications; 1958; 199-239.

28. McKenzie D. *The Infancy of Medicine*. London; 1927.

29. Diamond S, Dalessio DJ. Migraine headache. In: Diamond S, Dalessio DJ (eds). *The Practicing Physician's Approach to Headache*, 5th edition. Baltimore: Williams & Wilkins; 1992; 51-79.

30. Ross WD, McNaughton FL. Objective personality studies in migraine by means of the Rorschach method. *Psychosom Med J*. 1945; 2:23.

31. Sternbach R, Dalessio DJ, Kunzel M, Bowman G. MMPI patterns in common headache disorders. *Headache*. 1980; 20:311-315.

32. Kail AC. *The Medical Mind of Shakespeare*. Balgowlah, Australia: Williams & Wilkins; 1986; 236-237.

33. Browne AC. *Early American Herb Recipes*. New York: Crown; 1968.

34. Spence L. *An Encyclopedia of Occultism*. New York: University Books; 1960; 153.

35. Knapp RD Jr. Reports from the past 2. *Headache*. 1963; 3:112-122.

36. Isler H. Thomas Willis' two chapters on headache of 1672: A first attempt to apply the "new science" to this topic. *Headache*.1986; 26:95-98.

37. Critchley M. Migraine: From Cappadocia to Queen Square. *Background to Migraine*. London: Heinemann; 1969.

38. Cervantes M. *Don Quixote de la Mancha*.

39. World Federation of Neurology. Definition of migraine. In: Cochrane AL, ed *Background to Migraine*. London: Heinemann; 1970; 181-182.

40. Wolff HG. In: *Headache and Other Head Pain*, 2nd edition. New York: Oxford University Press; 1963.

41. Lauritzen M, Olesen J. Regional cerebral blood flow during migraine attacks by Xenon-133 inhalation and emission tomography. *Brain*. 1984; 107:447-461.

42. Olesen J, Larsen B, Lauritzen M. Focal hyperemia followed by spreading oligemia and impaired activation of rCBF in classic migraine. *Ann Neurol.* 1981; 9:344-352.

43. Skyhøj Olsen T, Friberg L, Lassen NA. Ischemia may be the primary cause of the neurological deficits in classic migraine. *Arch Neurol.* 1987; 44:156-161.

44. Weiller C, May A, Limmroth V, Juptner M, Kaube H, Schayck RV, et al. Brain stem activation in spontaneous human migraine attacks. *Nature Medicine.* 1995; 1:658-660.

45. Padover SK. *A Jefferson Profile.* New York: Day; 1956.

46. Pickering GW. *Creative Malady.* London: Oxford; 1974

47. Lippmann CW. Certain hallucinations peculiar to migraine. *J Nerv Ment Dis.* 1952; 116:346-351.

48. Todd J. The syndrome of Alice in Wonderland. *Can Med Assoc J.* 1955; 73:701-704.66

49. De Chirico G., Crosland M (translator). *Memoirs of Georgio de Chirico.* Philadelphia: Da Capo Press, 1994.

50. De Chirico G, Ashberry J (translator). *Hebdomeros.* Cambridge, MA: 1993.

51. Capra F. *The Name Above the Title.* New York: Macmillan; 1971.

52. Diamond S, Medina JL. Cluster headache variant: The spectrum of a new syndrome and its response to indomethacin. *Arch Neurol.* 1981; 38:705-709.

53. *Bibliotheca, Anatomica, Medica, Chirurgica, Etc,* volume 2. London; 1712; 351-369.

54. Critchley M. Bygone remedies for migraine. *Headache Q.* 1991; 2:171-176.

55. Jack DB. One hundred years of aspirin. *Lancet.* 1997; 350:437-439.

56. Fordyce J. *De Hemicrania;* 1758.

57. Liveing E. *On Megrim, Sich Headache and Some Allied Disorders.* London: J & A Churchill; 1873.

58. Symonds JA. Goulstonian lectures on "headache." *Med Times Gas.* 1858; 498.

59. Osler W. *Principles and Practice of Medicine,* 9th edition; 1912.

60. McFeely WS. *Grant – A Biography.* New York: WW Norton; 1982; 217-218.